Professional and Ethical Issues in Nursing

For Elsevier:

Commissioning Editor: Susan Young
Development Editor: Catherine Jackson
Project Manager: Jane Dingwall
Design Direction: Judith Wright

Professional and Ethical Issues in Nursing

Philip Burnard PhD MSc RGN RMN DipN CertEd RNT

Professor and Vice Dean, School of Nursing and Midwifery Studies, University of Wales College of Medicine, Cardiff, UK

Christine Chapman CBE BSc(Hons) MPhil SRN SCM RNT FRCN

Emeritus Professor of Nursing Education, School of Nursing and Midwifery Studies, University of Wales College of Medicine, Cardiff, UK

Editorial Consultant

Suzan Smallman RSCN RGN LLB(Hons) NDNCert

Formerly Professional Officer, Paediatrics and Community Nursing, Nursing and Midwifery Council, London, UK

THIRD EDITION

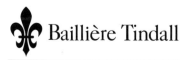 Baillière Tindall

EDINBURGH LONDON NEW YORK OXFORD PHILADELPHIA
ST LOUIS SYDNEY TORONTO 2004

BAILLIÈRE TINDALL
An imprint of Elsevier Limited

First published 1993
  Reprinted 1994, 1995, 1999, 2000, 2004, 2005

ISBN 0 7020 2685 9

British Library Cataloguing in Publication Data
A catalogue record for this book is available from the British Library

Library of Congress Cataloging in Publication Data
A catalog record for this book is available from the Library of Congress

ELSEVIER your source for books,
journals and multimedia
in the health sciences
www.elsevierhealth.com

Working together to grow
libraries in developing countries

www.elsevier.com | www.bookaid.org | www.sabre.org

ELSEVIER   BOOK AID
International   Sabre Foundation

The
publisher's
policy is to use
paper manufactured
from sustainable forests

Printed in China

Contents

PREFACE

In 1988, we published the first edition of this guide to professional and ethical issues in nursing. Since that time, the UKCC has updated and revised its Code of Professional Conduct twice and in 2002 its successor, the Nursing and Midwifery Council issued its first Code. The International Council of Nurses has also re-issued, for the first time in 27 years, a Code of Ethics for Nurses (2000). In addition, over the years, nursing and society have undergone changes. It is therefore time for a new edition of the book.

The present Code of Professional Conduct not only includes most of the material from the previous codes but also much that was in the UKCC's publication, *The Scope of Professional Practice*. This has meant that while the format of this book remains the same, the contents are ordered differently. In addition, new material, resulting from some well-publicised medical inquiries, has been included. Perhaps the biggest change that has occurred since the first edition is the increasing involvement of patients and their relatives in decision making, and this is reflected in the discussion of the issues.

The original authors have had the benefit of Suzan Smallman as consultant. She chaired the NMC group that produced the Code and therefore has intimate knowledge of the background affecting its formulation. We acknowledge her contribution.

As previously, each chapter examines a section of the Code and explores the concepts and problems that relate to it. We do not suggest that what is discussed on each issue is exhaustive, but we hope that it may serve as a catalyst to debate.

The breadth of debate is influenced by the perceptions of the authors, which in many ways are very different: male and female, married and single, sociologist and psychologist, general nursing and psychiatric nursing, Christian and searcher. However, what we have in common is that we are both nurses and deeply concerned with the standards of care offered to the public and to the development of the profession.

Previous editions of this book have been well received and it is hoped that this edition will be equally useful to a wide range of nurses, midwives and health visitors and other healthcare workers, in whatever setting they find themselves employed. As we have already stated, we do not claim to have definitive answers (in the ethical field they rarely exist), but we do hope to stimulate discussion.

Philip Burnard
Christine Chapman

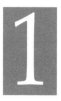 # Introduction

PROFESSIONAL AND ETHICAL ISSUES

This book is all about ethical and professional issues in nursing. Both of these areas are addressed by the Code of Professional Conduct. The introduction to the Code makes it clear that the main functions of the Code are, firstly, to inform the professions of the standards of professional conduct required of them in the exercise of their professional accountability and practice; secondly, to inform the public, employers and others of the standards that they can expect from registered practitioners; and thirdly, to make clear the responsibility of a registered practitioner to protect individuals and communities and the need to give safe and competent care. These points summarise the main thrust of the Code, which will be discussed in detail in subsequent chapters.

WHAT IS A PROFESSION?

Living languages, like living people, constantly change; they develop, become more sophisticated, sometimes decay and may be abused. The word 'profession' is an example of the dynamic activity affecting words. At one time, to be a member of a profession meant that one was either a member of the clergy, a physician or a lawyer; now it frequently means that the occupation so designated is one requiring a degree of skill and/or specific knowledge. So we have professional footballers as well as professional architects and engineers.

In an early attempt to overcome the lack of a succinct definition of the word 'profession', Carr-Saunders and Wilson (1964) stated:

> *the term profession ... clearly stands for something.*
> *That something is a complex of characteristics.*

Unfortunately, this statement does not help a great deal, as there is an absence of agreement as to what those characteristics are. Most lists of attributes, however, contain the following ideas:

> *A body of specific knowledge based on research.*

For many years, nurses were reluctant to claim a specific body of knowledge. However if, as Hockey (1974) asserts, nursing is a 'unique mix of knowledge and skills, many of which originated in other disciplines', then it may be said that nursing has a body of knowledge. Much of what nurses do has a theoretical basis which is rarely recognised. For example, germ theory lies at the base of all aseptic nursing procedures: whether or not masks need to be worn; barrier nursing techniques; lotions used to cleanse the skin, and so on. The laws of thermodynamics and other related physical laws underpin procedures such as temperature taking, tepid sponging and the care of the hypothermic patient. Psychological theories have affected views on allowing children to visit parents in hospital; the relationship between information, anxiety and pain; talking to the dying patient and the support given to bereaved relatives. Physiological theories should assist in the way medication is given; assist the patient with elimination; affect mobilisation after surgery and many other activities. Sociological theories contribute to the understanding of the role of the patient and nurse; how organisations function; patterns of power and other social factors. These are just examples of theories developed in a specific discipline contributing to nursing knowledge.

The qualifying statement 'based on research' has become more of a reality in the past decade, and as the testing of many traditional practices and knowledge increases so there is the excitement of discovering new knowledge and new ways in which it may be applied.

> *The amount and type of knowledge passed on to new entrants to a profession and the specific skills required are directed by members of that profession and the institutions involved in that education are validated by the profession.*

This is certainly the case in nursing, as both the content of educational programmes and the educational institutions in which they are taught have to be approved by the statutory bodies which register the successful students. Most professions maintain a register of licensed practitioners and the Nursing and Midwifery Council performs that function for nurses and midwives. The function of the register is to convey to the public that the registered practitioner has not only reached a satisfactory level of competence but also that a certain standard of behaviour can be expected. This latter point is exemplified in the next characteristic.

> *The attitude of the professional towards the client is one of service on an individual basis, the client's needs being placed before those of the professional.*

In that the knowledge and skills possessed by the professional may be relatively difficult for the client to access, there has to be an element of trust placed by the client in the professional, which in turn, the professional is prepared to accept. In order to assure the client as to the standards of behaviour that can be expected, some professions have a code of professional conduct. Deviation from this code may result in the professional's name being removed from the register of licensed practitioners.

The acceptable standard of practice is judged by fellow professionals, and only they are able to make decisions as to whether the quality of service is appropriate.

However, Etzioni (1969) states:

> *...the ultimate justification of a professional act is that it is to the best of the professional's knowledge, the right act.*

This demonstrates the high level of accountability and autonomy the professional must assume for professional practice.

Public recognition is important to the professional and the phrase, 'he's a real professional', is often used to indicate admiration of the skill demonstrated by an individual in a specific sphere of activity. The problem is that many people demonstrate a high level of skill in their job (consider the skill of a diamond cutter or a cabinet maker), yet these occupations are not normally considered to be professions. The level and type of knowledge underlying the skill and the relationship of the professional with the client are of a different order to that of a tradesman.

Professions tend to develop their own sub-culture. Greenwood (1957) describes this as 'consciousness of kind', which bands members together. This may be demonstrated by the formation of a professional organisation which not only facilitates this coming together for mutual help and support but also, according to Greenwood, allows members to 'learn and evaluate innovations in theory'. This provides a mutually stimulating milieu that is in marked contrast to the milieu of the non-professional.

Such a list does not answer the question, when is an occupation a profession? If an occupation is measured against such a list, how many positive 'ticks' are needed for the occupation to be called a profession? How many entitle it to be called a semi-profession?

Where is the cut-off point?

As already stated, as far as the proverbial man in the street is concerned, it is the certainty of a particular type of behaviour that earns a person the right to be called a 'professional', rather than the possession by that occupational group of any number of characteristics.

It is for this reason that groups, recognised or not as professions, adopt codes of conduct by which members can be guided in their behaviour. Some codes are very old, an example being the Hippocratic Oath, variants of which are still taken by graduating medical practitioners. Others, such as the Nursing and Midwifery Code of Conduct, are relatively new.

What is a code of conduct, and what is its purpose and standing? What it is not, is law. This may come as a surprise to many people, especially as in many professions a code of conduct is used to judge professional behaviour and may be cited in disciplinary committees. A code of conduct is what it says it is – a code or guide regarding appropriate behaviour for a specific group of people carrying out specific actions. Many codes of conduct claim to be based on ethical principles (e.g. ICN Code for Nurses, 1973); others do not overtly make this claim but nevertheless have ethically-based statements within their pages.

WHAT IS AN ETHICAL ISSUE?

The definition of ethics, is, like that of the word 'profession', fraught with difficulty. The Concise Oxford Dictionary states that it is the 'science of morals', which raises the question, what is meant by morals? Tschudin (1986) claims that 'ethics is caring', and that 'to act ethically is to care... to care for ourselves and others'. This approach is certainly attractive to those who claim to be members of caring professions. However, in a sense this is tautological and gives no real practical guide for action. Indeed, advocates for euthanasia often justify their claims to the right to end life on the basis that they are demonstrating 'care' and wish to relieve suffering, yet many would question whether such action is ethical. In place of the word 'ethical', many people would like to substitute the word 'right'. And it is the consideration of actions, beliefs and attitudes that make up the study of moral philosophy. In an attempt to decide what is 'right', 'good' and 'just', and to identify the difference between ethics and morals, Campbell (1979) acknowledged that the Greek and Latin from which the words derive mean roughly the same thing, 'that which is customary or generally accepted', but then went on to use the word 'morals' to describe the phenomena which are studied by 'ethics'.

The study of ethics may, therefore, be said to have two aspects. The first is related to how people 'should' behave and is based on the age-old debate engaged in by philosophers as to what is good, right and just. The second aspect, which can almost be considered to be the obverse of the same coin, is related to what people actually do and the pressures (personal, cultural and organisational) which influence their action. The first consideration may lead to statements, which ignore the consequences; the second sees the result of action as the most important factor. In making an ethical decision or drawing up a code of conduct, both aspects need to be considered.

Thiroux (1995) established a set of principles of ethics, which may be applied to any situation. They are:

1   The value of life

2   Goodness or rightness

3   Justice or fairness

4   Truth telling or honesty

5   Individual freedom.

It is important, according to Thiroux, to consider each of these principles when deciding on action. For example, if it is agreed that life is of supreme value, then when is it appropriate to stop striving to maintain it? When is death a realistic option? This is the first principle because without it the others are meaningless. However, Thiroux also states 'human beings should revere life and accept death', which may help in making the decision to turn off a life-support system. It may also remind the nurse that quality of life has to be considered as well as quantity. Yet this fact produces yet another dilemma. The quality of life enjoyed by a severely handicapped person may, to a young, healthy observer, appear to be very low indeed. To the person concerned, life may be very precious and worth living despite its restrictions.

The question as to the 'goodness' of an action has been debated since Aristotle, with a variety of measures being suggested by which an action may be judged. These range from original intention to the outcome of the activity.

Aristotle (see Chase, 1925) claimed that virtue lay in the appropriateness of the object or person for the task, so a 'good' knife is one that is sharp and cuts cleanly, because cutting is the function of a knife. It may also be aesthetically pleasing to look at, or it may be ugly, valuable or of little intrinsic worth, but if it does its job then it is 'good' and produces satisfaction or happiness. At first sight this is an attractive definition and may appear to solve the problem, but closer consideration will reveal some startling difficulties. What, for example, is the purpose of an individual? And can a person be described as 'good' because that purpose is met? The shorter Scottish Catechism states that the 'the chief aim of man is to glorify God and to enjoy Him forever', and Benjamin Disraeli stated that 'man... is born to believe'. Whether or not you agree with these statements, or whether you prefer to substitute other functions as the purpose of existence of human beings, it is easy to see that there may be individuals, perhaps physically or mentally handicapped, or aged and infirm, who are not able to perform the agreed function. Does this fact make them evil? Obviously not, so while the ability to function appropriately may be a useful way of assessing the value of a knife, it is no help in discussing the value of a man or a woman.

Many people would say that everyone knows what is 'right' and 'good' by the way in which their conscience acts, making them feel that something should, or should not, be carried out.

This is not a new idea. Bishop Butler, writing in 1736, developed an elaborate theory of conscience in which he claimed that having and obeying a conscience was essential to being classified as a human. He explained this by comparing the human personality with a watch, whose separate parts are only of use when placed in relationship to each another. Conscience, he claimed, was an essential part of the mechanism of the human personality and without it the individual was incomplete. Further, he claimed that an individual was motivated by three factors. Firstly, by 'particular passions' – that is, by basic drives such as hunger, some emotional reactions like fear and anger, and 'traits' like shyness and aggression. Secondly, by 'rational calculating principles', which calculate the individual's own long-term happiness, or what Butler called, 'cool self-love', and the calculation of the happiness of others, which he described as 'the principle of benevolence'. Thirdly, 'conscience', which would hold the superior position and enable the individual to decide between the rightness of an action under the other moderating forces. For an individual to disobey his or her conscience, according to Butler, was to destroy the natural balance of his or her personality.

All this sounds fine, but people do not always obey their conscience. Another difficulty is that my conscience may say one thing and, in an identical situation, yours may dictate another. Indeed, it is this very conflict which causes so many problems in nursing/medical practice. One person fully believes that it is wrong to destroy life in any circumstances, and therefore their conscience forbids them to assist with abortion; another believes, equally vehemently, that there are occasions when abortion is appropriate. Both must follow their conscience and thus no consensus can be reached. Instead, to use Sartre's (1948) words, 'the individual is entirely alone and abandoned in his decision; he and he alone must take the responsibility'. Such a view cannot therefore be the basis of a code of practice to be followed by a group of people, as each must make his/her own decision.

Another approach taken by a number of people when deciding on a course of action is to consider whether or not they would like it done to them. Charles Kingsley (1885) used this principle in his book *The Water Babies* when he created the character Mrs Do-as-you-would-be-done-by. Kant (1785) developed this point of view but also said that morality was doing one's duty for duty's sake. He described a series of actions as 'categorical imperatives'; that is, they must be followed. These are:

> *Act that the maxim of your action can become a universal law for all rational beings.*

> *Act as if the maxim of your action were to become by your will a universal law of nature.*

> *Act as to so treat humanity, whether in your own person or in that of any other, in every sense as an end, and never as a mere means.*

However, there are problems in applying this law of 'universality' when dealing with people who are themselves different and thus require different consideration. Does a commitment to preserve life mean that every patient who dies must be resuscitated, because that is the universal law? Some would argue 'yes', while many would want to say, 'it all depends'. Indeed, some would wish the patient to be given the opportunity to decide that resuscitation should or should not be carried out, for, if this choice is denied, the patient may be used as a 'means'. Denial of this choice may enable the nursing or medical staff to comfort themselves with the thought that everything had been done for the patient. Yet Kant said that the person must be an 'end in himself'. Consider the arguments used to support the decision to spend money on one area of healthcare rather than another; remarks such as 'he is so young' or 'she is too old and has had her life'; heart transplants before treatment for arthritis; acute care before chronic, and so on. In all these statements 'ends' are implied regarding the worth of the individual in relation to their likely contribution to society: means, not ends in themselves.

The consideration of whether or not an action produces happiness may be more acceptable. Philosophers known as Utilitarians, who may be represented by Jeremy Bentham and John Stuart Mill, assert that what is good is pleasure and happiness and that what is bad is pain. A good action, therefore, is one that produces more pleasure than pain. However, as any parent will know, a child's wish may have to be denied, thus producing unhappiness, because granting the request might be dangerous for the child. Can such denial be considered 'bad'? A further problem is that happiness for one group of people may produce unhappiness for another. Who, then, is satisfied? The group with most power? So develops the tyranny of the majority.

From this discussion, it is obvious that it is difficult (perhaps impossible) to formulate one rule by which every situation may be judged, so that it can be said, with certainty, that 'this action is good, right and just'. One common thread running through the debate is the conviction that people cannot be treated as a collection of things, such as knives, and that each person has to be regarded individually. Indeed, this is one of the first lessons to be learnt by any new entrant to a caring profession – all patients must be treated as individuals and yet all must be treated alike.

Even this statement may be contentious: discussion as to whether an action is just or fair cannot stop at saying that all must be treated alike when it is quite clear that all are not the same to start with. Is discrimination, either positive or negative, ever justified? We have already considered the problem in relation to expenditure on healthcare for specific groups. There is an apparent paradox in the statements, 'all people must be treated alike', and 'each person must be treated as an individual'. This paradox can be easily resolved: the nurse must not differentiate between patients on the grounds of colour, race, social class, education, attractiveness of personality and so on, but only on the basis of the activity required to meet the patient's individual needs. However, this does not help solve the dilemma as to how to allocate scarce resources.

Schrock (1980) claims that nurses are often less than honest in their dealings with patients, yet honesty and truthfulness make up Thiroux's fourth principle. Most people in everyday life support varying degrees of honesty and truth telling. So much is this accepted that the telling of a 'white lie' carries very little stigma, on the basis that to do so may be kind. Can this ever really be justified? To what extent is the 'whole truth' necessary? These are difficult questions, especially when caring for some patients, but they nevertheless involve a principle of morality.

Another aspect of morality relates to the use of equipment and time. Both are easily misappropriated and thus the employer is defrauded. Yet how often is this action considered stealing?

Thiroux's last principle is that of individual freedom. This, if present, will influence the way the first four principles are held and acted upon. What is more, it implies autonomy of action so that no one else can be held responsible for the actions of another. Nurses frequently question to what extent they have autonomy, and, therefore, whether they can be held responsible for the care they give. Codes of conduct assume that the individual is accountable. To what extent are they correct when a professional is employed in a bureaucratic structure?

What all this apparently leads to is a belief that a moral basis for action has to be rooted in the perception of the intrinsic worth of the individual and that person's right to self-determination. (Christians would back up this respect by explaining that man is created in the image of God.) The debate as to what constitutes a person has already been touched upon. Most agree that it includes an individual with humanoid characteristics, with a capacity, however small, to communicate and to be communicated with (not necessarily by speech). 'Respect of person' in this context requires activity which is a combination of both rational and emotional elements, used in a relationship of involvement with other individuals, so that their wishes, thoughts and aspirations are taken into account.

This approach, the respect of individuals, has some important implications. First, there is no final set of moral rules to guide every action: modification may have to take place depending upon the individual. Secondly, the individual is given greater value than society. Thirdly, it demands an attempt to maintain an ongoing relationship with the individual, so that the person does not become an object to whom things are done. These factors are costly in time, resources and human endeavour and do not provide quick and easy answers.

It is in the light of this type of discussion that the United Kingdom Central Council for Nursing, Midwifery and Health Visiting (UKCC) issued, not a set of rules, but the first *Code of Professional Conduct* (1983) as guidance for registered practitioners. The Code was revised on three occasions, taking into account comments from those using it. The provision of the Code was not welcomed by all. Some of the displeasure was due to misunderstanding of its function, fear that it might become a stick with which to beat the profession, and concern that it might be unrealistic in its demands. The UKCC stated that the aims of the code were to:

> *...establish and improve standards of training and professional conduct ... and the provision of advice for nurses, midwives and health visitors on standards of professional conduct.*

Eventually it was felt that some aspects of the Code required elaboration and so the UKCC published a paper called *The Scope of Professional Practice* (1992) in which they outlined the way the profession might develop and the way in which nurses might enlarge their role. The principles were drawn from the Code, and stated that the registered nurse, midwife and health visitor must:

- Be satisfied that each aspect of practice is directed to meeting the needs and serving the interests of the patient or client

- Endeavour always to achieve, maintain and develop knowledge, skill and competence to respond to those needs and interests

- Honestly acknowledge any limits of personal knowledge and skill and take steps to remedy any relevant deficits in order effectively and appropriately to meet the needs of patients and clients

- Ensure that any enlargement or adjustment of the scope of personal professional practice must be achieved without compromising or fragmenting existing aspects of professional practice and care and that the requirements of the Council's Code of Professional Conduct are satisfied throughout the whole area of practice

- Recognise and honour the direct or indirect personal accountability borne for all aspects of professional practice

- In serving the interests of patients and clients and the wider interests of society, avoid any inappropriate delegation to others which compromises those interests.

In 2002 the Nursing and Midwifery Council, the successor to the UKCC, issued a fresh code in which they endeavoured to include the intent of both the UKCC code and the points in *The Scope of Professional Practice*. This is printed in full in Appendix 1. Although this code has differences in the order of the items and some of the wording is different, the intent of this new code is unchanged from those previously issued. All emphasise that the first consideration of the practitioner is the good of the patient and client.

Rumbold (1986) claims that professional codes serve three main functions:

1 To reassure the public

2 To provide guidelines for the profession to regulate and discipline its members

3 To provide a framework on which individual members can formulate decisions.

In the subsequent chapters we discuss the Code itself.

REFERENCES

Campbell AV. Moral dilemmas in medicine. Edinburgh: Churchill Livingstone, 1979

Carr-Saunders AM, Wilson PA. The professions. London: F Cass, 1964

Chase DP. Aristotle, Nichomachean Ethics. London: Dent, trans. 1925

Etzioni A (ed). The semi-professions and their organisation. New York: Free Press, 1969

Greenwood E. Attributes of a profession. Social Work 1957; 11(3): 45-53

Hockey L. Forschung un Bereich. Osterreiche Krankenpflege Zeitschrift 1974; 27(4): 41-43

International Council for Nurses. Code for Nurses. Geneva: ICN, 1973

Kant I. Fundamental principles of the metaphysics of morals. (Trans: Abbott TK). New York: Library of Literal Arts, 1785

Kingsley CC. The water babies. London: Garland, 1885

Mill JS. Utilitarianism. London: Longman, 1865

Nursing and Midwives Council. Code of Professional Conduct. London: NMC, 2002

Rumbold G. Ethics in nursing practice. London: Baillière Tindall, 1986

Sartre J-P. Existentialism and humanism. London: Methuen, 1948

Schrock R. A question of honesty in nursing practice. Journal of Advanced Nursing1980; 5(2): 135-148

Thiroux JP. Ethics, theory and practice. 5th edn. Englewood Cliffs, California: Prentice-Hall, 1995

Tschudin V. Ethics in nursing: the caring relationship. London: Heinemann, 1986

UKCC. Code of Professional Conduct. London: UKCC, 1983

UKCC. The Scope of Professional Practice. London: UKCC, 1992

2 Respect

How does a person become a patient? Apparently by the simple process of becoming ill. Yet sociologists argue that there are a variety of ways in which this status may be awarded. Talcott Parsons (1966) suggests that a person has the right to be called 'sick' only if competent help is sought and there is an active desire to get well, demonstrated by co-operation in the steps that are designed to assist a return to health. If these criteria are met then the person has the right to be excused other roles and to be designated 'sick'. Certainly this is the way society works, in that it demands certification by a medical practitioner if the indisposition lasts more than a few days and absence from work is requested.

Robinson (1971), however, showed in his study of families in Swansea that the presence of physical symptoms was not always sufficient to ensure that a person sought medical advice. Frequently, the difficulty of being excused social roles, the danger of losing a job if 'off sick', the problem of finding someone to care for children and other non-medical social factors, meant that the person deferred or sacrificed the right to be classified as 'sick' and failed to seek help.

Why does a person become a nurse? When prospective applicants are interviewed there are many reasons given, but at some point the applicant says something to the effect that they want to help care for people. Certainly, that is the image held by the public. A nurse is one who 'cares'. What is more, it is expected that this care will be of a personal nature; that is, the nurse will care for them, not just as a 'patient', but as an individual. Jourard (1971) put it like this:

> one of the events that we believe inspires hope in a patient is the conviction that someone cares about him.

If this is true then nurse/patient relationships are of prime importance.

Some definitions of nursing were discussed in Chapter 1. The Royal College of Nursing (2003) agreed the following definition of nursing:

> The use of clinical judgement in the provision of care to enable people to improve, maintain or recover health, to cope with health problems, and to achieve the best possible quality of life, whatever their disease or disability, until death.

What all these definitions have in common is that they focus on the individual client or patient, stressing the maintenance of health, the prevention of disease, and the aim of the individual's independence.

It is clear that the roles of nurse and patient are complimentary.

Without the presence of a patient there would be no need of a nurse (the word nurse in this context is used in its generic sense and therefore includes all branches of care provided by nurses).

The problem is that most nurses find themselves working in an organisation which may have other aims than that of fostering effective interpersonal relationships; this is true even of those who work outside traditional healthcare institutions. Melia (1981) found that most nurses were concerned with 'getting the work done' and it is often a fact that nurses are rewarded for bureaucratic efficiency rather than for the quality of the care they provide. This is in stark contrast to the guidance given in the Code, which enjoins the nurse to 'to promote and protect the interests and dignity of patients/clients'.

To be able to assess the interests of the patient or client the nurse has to have time to develop a personal relationship and to foster the feeling of empathy. The development of empathy requires the nurse to 'step into the shoes' of patients in order to perceive the world through their eyes and to feel what they feel. Armed with this knowledge the nurse has then to return to the role of nurse using the knowledge gained to enhance the care given. This requires the nurse to get involved with the patient, an activity that was frequently frowned upon in the past and is still regarded by some as 'unprofessional'. What is unprofessional and unethical is the impersonal approach which results in all patients being treated as if they were identical, which is clearly not so. Stan van Hooft (2003) states that

> *the elucidation of the caring perspective in ethics has*
> *encouraged proponents of the emotional concept of nurse*
> *caring to see such caring as morally excellent and as providing*
> *sufficient ethical justification for caring actions.*

It would be pleasing to feel that nursing has moved on from the observations of Jourard (1964) when he observed that

> *Much of contemporary interpersonal competence seems to entail success in getting patients to conform to the rules they are supposed to play in the social system of the hospital so that the system will work smoothly, work will get done faster and the patient will be less of a bother to care for.*

What an indictment of a group of people who apparently entered the profession to care for others! The problem in some cases is that the nurse's desire to give physical care is such that the patient is not allowed to return to 'independence' even though that is an important aspect of care. Talcott Parsons (1966), in defining the role of the patient, said that not only must the patient seek competent help and positively wish to recover, but also they must comply with the treatment offered. This may be appropriate, but in the final analysis the patient or client has the right to self-determination. It is difficult to accept that advice, offered with the patient's best interest in heart, may be disregarded or positively rejected. Perhaps the health educator has the most difficult position in this respect. It is disheartening when a patient with chronic respiratory disease continues to smoke, or the obese patient with a failing heart refuses to diet, but that is their right.

RIGHTS AND RESPONSIBILITIES

What the are the rights and responsibilities of nurses and patients when involved in patient care? Over the years the act of nursing has evolved from being a collection of tasks performed on a passive patient to a partnership between the nurse and the patient where both endeavour to achieve

Table 2.1 The four areas of responsibility of the nurse	
Patient's rights	**Nurse's duties**
Health or a peaceful death	To promote health
	To prevent illness
	To restore health
	To alleviate suffering

agreed healthcare goals. This implies assessment, goal setting, planned intervention and evaluation of progress. All this is dependent on effective communication and interaction, although the nurse may have to act where the patient has not the strength, knowledge or will to act independently.

The *ICN Code for Nurses* (ICN 2000) defined four main areas of responsibility for the nurse: to promote health, to prevent illness, to restore health and to alleviate suffering. However one person's right may become another person's duty (see Table 2.1).

Stockwell (1972) also found that patients felt that they had the right to receive:

1. Skilled care, 'a nurse you can depend upon'

2. Attention to 'trivial matters'

3. More information

4. More opportunity to voice worries and needs.

One of the responsibilities of the nurse is to act as the patient's advocate in situations where the patient is unable to

Table 2.2 Rights and responsibilities of nurse and patient

Nurse		Patient	
Rights to have	*Responsibilities to give*	*Rights to have*	*Responsibilities to give*
Experience	Skilled care	Skilled care	Cooperation
Recognition	Individual care	Individual care	Conform to routine
Reward	Information	Information	Gratitude
(status,	Emotional support	Empathy	
money,			
gratitude)			

independently. Advocacy is a frequently misunderstood concept. *The Concise Oxford Dictionary* defines an advocate as 'one who pleads or speaks for another'. Patients frequently find it difficult to fully express their needs and fears. The nurse who has cultivated the skill of empathy and who has frequent personal interaction with the patient may be able to interpret the patient's needs to others and to act as a go-between when other healthcare professionals appear, to the patient, to be unapproachable. The nurse may also be required to explain to the patient alternative lines of treatment and to ensure that the patient fully understands the implication of proposed treatment before consent is given. This does not absolve other healthcare professionals from their responsibility to act in the best interest of the patient and most will do so, but it does place the nurse, who has a close ongoing relationship with the patient, in a special position of responsibility. Brown (1985) claims that advocacy is a means of transferring power back to the patient.

The relationship may therefore be elaborated to show the rights and responsibilities on both sides (see Table 2.2).

Earned rights

Curtin and Flaherty (1982) offer another slant on this debate. They suggest that nurses have 'earned rights' by virtue of the work they do, their experience in caring for others and as a result of their education and training. Among the earned rights that they suggest that nurses have are the following:

1 The right to practice nursing in accord with professionally defined standards

2 The right to participate in and promote the growth and direction of the profession

3 The right to be trusted by members of the public

4 The right to intervene when necessary to protect patients, clients or members of the public

5 The right to testify authoritatively to the community about the healthcare needs of people

6 The right to be believed when speaking in their area of expertise

7 The right to be respected by those inside and outside the profession for their knowledge, abilities, experience and contributions

8 The right to be trusted by colleagues

9 The right to give and receive from colleagues support, guidance and correction

10 The right to be compensated fairly for services rendered.

In summary, Styles (1983), in her declaration of belief about the purpose and nature of nursing says:

> *I believe in nursing as a humanistic field in which the fullness,*
> *self-respect, self-determination and humanity of the nurse*
> *engage the fullness, self-respect, self-determination and*
> *humanity of the client.*

This is surely acting in the best interest of the patient and client.

EQUITY OF CARE

Justice would imply that all individuals, patients or clients, should be treated the same, but that denies their differences and individuality. We live in a multi-cultural society and the Code requires nurses to promote and protect the interests and dignity of patients and clients, irrespective of gender, age, race, ability, sexuality, economic status, life style, culture and religious or political beliefs (Paragraph 2.2). Account therefore has to be taken of a patient's customs.

Customs are a person's regular or established ways of behaving. They are often linked to that person's country of birth, to their upbringing, life experience and belief systems. For some, customs are so ingrained that they are carried out unconsciously; others (and particularly if they are linked to a particular spiritual belief or value system) are very precisely carried out with attention to ritual. Because customs of any sort are embedded so deeply in the background and experience of the individual it is important that the nurse respects individual differences, for to question a person's customs is to question the person's self-concept and detract from their dignity.

A problem arises here as to how nurses can recognise other people's customs. Sometimes the behaviour of other people, if it is unusual, may seem unintelligible or irrational. If this is the case, then it is easy to dismiss the person's customs as peculiar and possibly to interpret their behaviour as uncooperative. It is essential that nurses develop a background knowledge of a variety of customs that they may encounter and also that they understand and clarify their own customs and behaviour.

CUSTOMS

In order to develop an understanding of the variety of customs that relate to specific groups of people it is necessary to draw on a number of sources. A short list may include anthropology, geography, sociology, psychology and theology. Anthropology can help in placing people in a particular cultural and social situation (Fox 1975) and can aid in developing a deeper perspective on different styles and ways of living together in a particular country. Geography gives clues as to the way particular life styles are based in the physical world, for example life in mountainous areas or in low temperatures. Sociology offers an analysis and possible explanation of how and why people form groups, co-operate, and generally exist in a state of interdependence (Chapman 1977). Psychology offers a closer focus on the individual and suggests a variety of theories about the nature of individual thinking, feeling and behaving. It must be borne in mind that much sociological and psychological literature is Western in orientation. The degree to which Western thinking can readily accommodate cultural differences is open to question. Can a theorist working and thinking in the West truly understand and account for the thinking and behaviour of those living in the East?

Theology can explain some forms of behaviour and customs from a religious point of view. Again the temptation to view one's own interpretation of religion as the right one needs to be resisted when caring for patients whose belief is totally different. This does pose something of a problem. If a particular set of beliefs is felt to be 'true', then it is naturally difficult to accept that another set of beliefs may also be 'true'! The nurse must be able to acknowledge and accept such ambiguity when caring for patients and clients.

Each of these disciplines offers a different sort of analysis of human action. The skilled nurse would do well to consider these various perspectives as an aid to developing a rich background from which to view a patient's behaviour and customs. Human action never occurs in isolation; it is always embedded in the particular social and psychological context prevalent at the time. Ideas gained from these disciplines may also be used to enable nurses to clarify their own beliefs and customs. The questions that need to be answered are 'why do I act in the way I do?' and 'how did I come to adopt these patterns of behaviour?' To answer, some knowledge of the sociological concept of socialisation and of the psychological process known as introjection is needed. Reflection and introspection are also required.

Reflection

The first stage in the reflective process is becoming conscious of the fact that we act at all. This may seem a ludicrous statement – surely we all know that we act? A moment's reflection, however, will probably reveal that we do not often notice how we act. Much action is spontaneous and without forethought or attention. What is being suggested here is a willing and conscious attention to what is being done and why. Heron (1977) refers to this process as 'conscious use of the self'. Once a person begins to consciously notice what is being done, it is easier to identify the reasons for doing it.

Having begun this process of noticing, it is then possible to compare that action with the theories or explanations offered by the disciplines already mentioned. In this way the theories can be 'personalised'. This reflective and comparative process can lead to an enhanced degree of self-understanding, without which it is impossible to understand the behaviour and customs of others.

Values

The process of valuing or holding values consists, according to Raths, Harmin and Simon (1966) of three sub-processes: (a) prizing one's own beliefs and behaviours, (b) choosing those beliefs and behaviours and (c) acting upon them. Like customs, values are deeply grounded in cultural heritage, experience and personal belief systems. Also, like customs, they are part of a person's self-concept: and those valued or held to be important make the individual who they are. Values are things that modify behaviour through a process of self-monitoring. Personal value systems allow or disallow certain actions. As with customs, values vary from culture to culture, from group to group, and from person to person. It can never be assumed that other people's value systems are similar to one's own. Thus in nursing, respect for other people's values is vital.

The process of self-reflection and introspection can again help to identify our own values. An aid to this process is a series of exercises in value clarification offered by Simon, Howe and Kirschenbaum (1978). They argue that many people are unaware of their own value system and therefore have difficulty in knowing how to make decisions about how to act. Through clearly identifying our values we are better equipped to make decisions about how to live our lives and also to appreciate the differences between our value system and those of other people.

It is one thing to identify and clarify personal values and quite another to appreciate the effect that one's value system has on other people. Values are reflected in most of the things that are done and particularly in the way things are said. Thus there is a need to pay attention to our verbal behaviour in order that our value system does not offend other people. Consider, for instance, the following situations:

- The patient who tells you that they've 'no religion' when a nursing assessment is being made

- The patient with AIDS, who names his gay partner as next of kin

- The unmarried adolescent girl who is admitted with complications during pregnancy.

In each of these situations, what is said to the patient will reflect a particular value system. It is not possible to escape from the valuing process. For instance, it may be acknowledged in each of the above cases that the life situation of each person is perfectly acceptable. On the other hand, some or all of these life-styles may be unacceptable to the admitting nurse. Whether 'accepted' or not, a particular value statement is made. In this sense there is no neutral ground. What is important, however, is that there is an acknowledgement that whatever position is held, that of the other person is equally valid. A nurse is on difficult ground if condemning others for the values they hold, and on even more difficult ground if that condemnation is verbalised. Such behaviour is not in keeping with the Code of Professional Conduct, in treating the patient with dignity regardless of any external variation.

SPIRITUAL BELIEFS

Linked with the question of values is that of spiritual belief. In order for the nurse to consider thoughtfully other people's spiritual beliefs it is important that they appreciate the basic differences between various sorts of faith, indeed various ways of living, without a set of religious beliefs, such as atheism, agnosticism and secular humanism. Spiritual beliefs have been described as those concerned with personal meaning or how we make sense of the world around us (Burnard, 1987). That meaning may be framed in religious terms or not. The person who adopts an atheistic, agnostic or secular humanistic position is still creating meaning. It is just that such meaning does not include a concept of God. It is worth considering the basic tenets of the major religions of the world and the non-religious philosophies that enable people to create meaning.

Christianity

While Christianity can be divided into a number of major classes such as Orthodox, Protestant and Roman Catholic, there are also a variety of groupings within each division. Nevertheless, there are certain tenets of faith that are common to all. All major Christian churches believe in the historical figure of Jesus of Nazareth as the Son of God, born of a virgin. The essence of Christianity can be identified in the Apostle's Creed:

> *I believe in God the Father Almighty, Creator of Heaven and Earth and in Jesus Christ his only Son, our Lord who was conceived by the Holy Spirit, born of the Virgin Mary; suffered under Pontius Pilate, was crucified dead and buried, he descended into Hell: the third day he rose again and ascended*

*into Heaven: is seated on the right hand of God the Father
Almighty from thence he shall come to judge the quick and the
dead. I believe in the Holy Ghost: the holy Catholic Church; the
Communion of Saints: the forgiveness of sins: the resurrection
of the body: and the life of the world to come. Amen.*

The word Catholic in this passage refers to the notion of
universality and is not synonymous with the Roman Catholic
Church. Christians of all denominations (and a great many of
them are described by Sampson (1982), celebrate the
following festivals: Christmas, Lent, Good Friday, Easter
Sunday and Whitsun (Pentecost). However there are a
number of variations in practice in individual
denominations. It cannot be assumed that all Christians
believe the same, beyond the basic tenets identified above.
The theological and doctrinal position adopted by different
denominations varies greatly, as does the attention paid to
ritual and ceremony. These variations are vitally important
to individual believers and are well articulated by Sampson
(1982) and Rumbold (1986).

Judaism

Judaism is a religion essentially of a particular people, the
Jews. The history of Judaism and much of its theological
basis can be found in the Old Testament of the Holy Bible.
The law of the Jewish people is written in the Torah, or first
five books of the Old Testament. They await the coming of
the Messiah and do not recognise Jesus of Nazareth as the
Messiah. Important Jewish festivals include: Rosh Hashanah
(Jewish New Year), Yom Kippur (the Day of Atonement),
Succoth (Feast of Tabernacles), Simchath Torah (Rejoicing in
the Law), Chanukah (the Feast of Esther), Purim (the Feast of
Lots), Pesach (the Passover) and Tishah B'Av (Mourning for

the Destruction of the Temple). There are various groups, as in Christianity, and therefore the strictness of the way an individual observes the feasts will vary. Orthodox Jews require food to be prepared following a specific ritual (kosher) and will abstain from certain types of meat, notably pork.

Since the founding of the State of Israel Judaism has taken on a strong political element which often clouds its religious basis.

Hinduism

Hinduism is an ancient religion, originally centred in India and Nepal but which has spread wherever Indians have settled. Hindus believe in many gods, but also believe that all these are manifestations of one God. Hinduism has no fixed creed and is very diverse in the beliefs held. There are a variety of schools of Hindu philosophy and a number of separate religions have developed from it, including Buddhism. In the Hindu religion the cow is considered a sacred animal and therefore beef is not eaten.

Islam

Muslims follow the religion of Islam. Islam literally means submission and Muslims are committed to submitting themselves to the will of God. In the Islamic faith God is called Allah and Muslims believe him to be the one true God. The consider Mohammed to be the last great prophet following chronologically after the Jewish prophets and Jesus Christ, and they follow his teachings recorded in the Koran. Muslims also require animals used for food to be prepared in a ritual manner (Halal). Again there are different groupings of Muslims with some variety in belief. As with Judaism there is a strong political arm to the religion and some countries can be designated as Islamic States.

The recent events in the Middle East and of 11th September 2001 demonstrated the level of violence that some Muslims feel justified in using and the way in which they are prepared to sacrifice their own lives for their belief. This attitude is not universal and many Muslims condemn violence and deeply regret the way in which they have all been classified as terrorists.

Clearly, this cannot claim to be an exhaustive description of the religions mentioned nor is it comprehensive of all the world's beliefs. There is considerable literature on these topics to which the reader is referred. It is important, in this context, to note the considerable variations that different cultures give to religious experience and observation.

Finally, we may consider the issues of atheism and agnosticism. Both can be seen as a dimension of spirituality, in that both are aspects of a person's belief system and an attempt to create meaning. Both should therefore be respected.

Atheism

Atheism is the unequivocal denial of the possibility of the existence of God. The atheist is the 'unbeliever'. It is interesting to ponder on an individual reaction to such a position. For instance, it is possible to respond by seeing the person as 'wrong', or that the person just needs further reflection or clarification or more education to bring them to the truth. Or can they be accepted as they are? Various reactions are possible: the least acceptable is the notion that somehow the believer is 'right' and the unbeliever is 'wrong'. Belief in God must necessarily involve a 'leap of faith' (Kierkegaard, 1959). There is no ultimate scientific proof in the existence or non-existence of God. Individuals either do or do not believe. Neither does the absence of belief necessarily preclude any sort of moral position. An unbeliever is quite as able to lead a moral life as a believer. Indeed Simone de Beauvoir argued that unbelievers had to lead a 'more moral' life than believers as there was no final arbiter of right and wrong for unbelievers – they were necessarily thrown back on their own decision-making as a guide to conduct. The believer can be 'forgiven'; the unbeliever has to forgive himself.

The atheist has to look beyond the concept of God for meaning. That they have to do that does not mean that they do not have spiritual needs. The spiritual needs of the atheist (in terms of a search for meaning) are just as vital as they are for believers. Some atheists find a sense of meaning in secular humanism. The base argument of secular humanism is that outlined by Blackman (1968). Briefly, the argument is this: people are alone in that there is no God. Because they are alone, they are responsible for themselves. They also have a joint responsibility for all other persons. In acting for themselves they should act as if acting for all mankind. To do less than this is selfishness, and not, so Blackman argues, secular humanism. Such a philosophy offers a sense of meaning; the atheist is responsible for himself and for others. As a result the 'golden rule' applies, 'treat others as you would wish to be treated'. This then, is the basis for morality and for meaning without recourse to belief in God.

Agnosticism

The agnostic, on the other hand, is in a slightly different position, arguing that, because it is impossible to prove or disprove the existence of God, silence on the issue is the only wise move (Bullock & Stallybrass, 1977). The agnostic is neither a believer nor an unbeliever; he holds the view that discussion about the matter is misplaced, because such an issue can only be a matter of faith. Again, such a position does not rule out the need for meaning or morality. The agnostic, like the atheist, still needs to discover or invest life with meaning in order to know how to live. Some may argue that the only meaning that can be found in life is that which individuals invest in it (Kopp, 1972). In other words, there is no ultimate meaning for the way things are; people bring meaning to their actions. Meaning, therefore, is an intrinsic concept and dependent on the individual's reasoning or perception.

These are thumbnail sketches of two positions alternative to that of a belief in God. There are, of course, other positions, such as that of the person who does not know whether or not he believes in God, or the person who does not think such issues are important.

There are many situations in nursing when these issues need to be considered. As we have already noted, on admission the question of the patient's religion is raised. Such a question makes an assumption that the person is a 'believer'. Indeed, it is quite possible that many patients, faced with such a question and uncertain of their beliefs, will say 'Church of England' or 'Catholic', whether or not they are really members of those churches, in order not to embarrass themselves. It may take considerable bravery to answer 'none' or 'atheist'. We need to think hard about how we pose such questions.

Also, it is necessary to consider the sort of value judgements nurses make regarding other people's belief systems. If the nurse is a 'believer', is there likely to be a harsh judgement of the 'unbeliever'? If, on the other hand, the nurse is an 'unbeliever', is the patient's belief dismissed? It is important to acknowledge that the patient's belief system may not coincide with that of the nurse. Nor is it appropriate that the nurse evangelises or proselytises for either position. Nurses in the role of carer are not required to convert others to belief or unbelief.

There are other delicate issues that may arise. For example, the unbeliever may not feel the need for a conventional funeral service. Secular forms of service are available through national secular services. Not all unbelievers dread death, nor need it be a fearful event for unbelieving relatives.

It would be a great disservice to a variety of ways of addressing spiritual matters if the term 'spiritual' was only understood as being concerned with religious matters. Nurses need to be open minded about this important aspect of nursing care.

Finally, David Cooper (1992) offers a useful list of dos and don'ts regarding the care of patients from various cultures, which can be found in Appendix 2.

GENETICS AND NURSING

The increasing understanding of the genetic make-up of individuals has led to techniques that give rise to major social, ethical and legal problems. The pressure towards testing individuals to determine whether they carry genes specific to certain diseases may give rise to stigma and discrimination. Some people may be seen as less worthy of treatment and care because of their inherited situation. Misuse of genetic data could also lead to racism and lack of respect for certain populations. It is important that the nurse does not fall into the trap of considering individuals as merely a collection of genes.

The nurse needs to understand the issues involved and be prepared to ensure that patients have adequate information and counselling before embarking on genetic testing. Testing should remain voluntary and should only be carried out with informed consent. The results must also be confidential to the individual so that at all times their dignity is maintained.

The suggestion that humans may be cloned is rejected by all health professionals. The World Health Professions Association, which is an alliance of the International Council of Nurses, the International Pharmaceutical Federation and the World Medical Association, has stated publicly (2002) its opposition to the cloning of human beings and has called for a global ban on further experimentation.

Professional boundaries

People can be vulnerable for many reasons but certainly when someone experiences ill health their vulnerability increases, particularly when they find themselves in an unusual setting, such as a hospital. At this time the patient puts their trust in those caring for them such as the nurse. Nurses must never breech this trust by abusing the patient in any way. Abuse can take many forms – physical, psychological, verbal or sexual. None is acceptable behaviour.

The nurse generally holds the position of power in the relationship with the patient and she must ensure that the relationship is appropriate at all times. This relationship must be based on safeguarding the interests and healthcare needs of the patient.

The professional boundary is defined as the limits of behaviour, which allow the nurse and the patient to engage in a therapeutic caring relationship. This relationship should be based upon trust, respect and the appropriate use of power and should not be used by the nurse to establish social or personal contacts.

Conscientious objection

Just as patients and clients have different beliefs and practices, so do staff, and it is a fundamental right of any person in the UK to exclude themselves from any specific procedure or situation on 'conscientious' grounds. Even in wartime, a person who objects to killing may request exemption from military service. There is an important distinction to be made between the person who objects to an action because of strongly held and soundly based principles and the person who objects at a specific time because of a conflict of professional judgement. For example, it may be possible for a nurse to accept that in certain situations patients may benefit from electro-convulsive therapy, but on a specific occasion to consider that the patient is too physically frail to receive such treatment. In this case, although the objection is made on professional grounds, the medical staff in charge of the case may not accept the objection as valid. Quite a different situation would exist if the nurse objected to the treatment on the grounds that it was morally wrong because it interfered with the normal functioning of the brain. In this case it would be appropriate for the nurse to be relieved from participation in the treatment on conscientious grounds.

Obviously such objections based on principle will be known in advance of the treatment and the nurse should make her objection known so that appropriate staffing arrangements may be made to ensure that the patient has adequate care. The bases for such principles may be religious or moral and as such cannot be the subject of rules.

Categorical imperatives

The philosopher Kant (1785) endeavoured to lay down guidance for individuals who faced the difficult situation of having to decide on the rightness or otherwise of a course of action. He called his guidelines 'categorical imperatives' thus giving them more strength than perhaps many would accord them. The first of these imperatives states that a person should:

Act only on that maxim through which you can at the same time will that it should become a universal law.

It is this type of action, based on a fundamental principle, that forms the ground for conscientious objection. However it is also expected that the nurse will act in such a way that no harm will befall the patent. Therefore it is both morally expected and, to a degree, required by law that a nurse should make clear any reasons that may exist which indicate to her that a proposed course of treatment will not only be of little benefit but may also be harmful to the patient.

It is this type of action that may result in disagreement between healthcare professionals and which, in an ideal world, would be resolved by open and frank discussion. However, this is not an ideal world and if the treatment ordered is the responsibility of another professional, then the nurse may fail to halt its progress. In such a case it would be wise of the nurse to record the objection made and the grounds for dissent. Such a decision is one for the individual to take and is not one that can be resolved by resort to hierarchical power or policy statements; nevertheless the nurse making the objection may be required to justify the action taken.

In 1985 the National Board for Nursing, Midwifery and Health Visiting for Scotland issued a Guidance Paper for nurses who object to medical treatment. In it they suggested that the following steps might be helpful:

> *The person who issued the instructions should be asked for clarification.*
>
> *The nurse expressing concern should provide factual, rationally defensible evidence for her concern.*
>
> *Clearly documented nursing assessments and records are essential.*

Any form of conscientious objection demands that the nurse is able to identify and understand her own value and belief system, why her beliefs are held and their possible limitations, and the areas of possible conflict with others. Without such self-awareness and clarification, decisions of conscience may be made 'blindly' and without rational thought. It is important in a professional context that objections are not made on a whim but are firmly grounded in rational thought.

Verbalising objections

It is important that all nurses who wish to object are able to express their objection clearly and to verbalise it appropriately. Such expression may be advanced by the nurse developing assertion skills (Alberti & Emmons, 1982). Assertiveness enables a person to be clear about what they wish to say and to develop the courage to say it clearly and if necessary repeat it several times. In the past the nursing profession has tended to produce compliant individuals. The hierarchical nature of the medical profession and the perceived lower status of the nurse enhanced this subservient self-image. However both nursing and medicine have changed and although there may be individuals who cling to the old, traditional view, most healthcare professionals recognise the important, if different, roles that they each play, and there is a much greater sense of working as a team.

■ QUESTIONS FOR REFLECTION AND DISCUSSION

1 What factors make it difficult for you to form a therapeutic relationship?

2 Are there any circumstances that would make it difficult for you to care for a patient?

REFERENCES

Alberti RE, Emmons MI. Your perfect right: a guide to assertive living. 4th ed. San Louis, California: Impact Publishers , 1982

Blackman HJ. Humanism. Harmondsworth: Pelican, 1968

Brown M. Matter of commitment. Nursing Times 1984; 61 (18): 26-27

Bullock A, Stallybrass O (eds). The Fontana dictionary of modern thought. London: Fontana, 1977

Burnard P. Spiritual distress and the nursing response: theoretical considerations and counselling skills. Journal of Advanced Nursing 1978; 12: 377-382

Chapman CM. Sociology for nurses. London: Baillière Tindall, 1977

Cooper DB. Transcultural issues and approaches. In: Wright H, Giddey M (eds) Mental health nursing: from first principles to professional practice. London: Chapman Hall, 1993

Curtin L, Flaherty M. Nursing ethics: theories and pragmatics. Englewood Cliffs, New Jersey: Prentice Hall, 1982

Fox F. Encounter with anthropology. Harmondsworth: Penguin, 1975

Heron J. Behavioural analysis in education and training. Human potential research project. University of Guildford, 1977

International Council for Nurses. Code for Nurses. Geneva: ICN, 2000

Jourard SM. The transparent self. New York: Van Nostrand, 1964

Jourard SM. The transparent self. 2nd ed. New York: Van Nostrand, 1971

Kant I. Fundamental principles of metaphysics of morals (trans Abbott TK). New York: Library of Literal Arts, 1785

Kierkegaard S. Either/or. Vol.1. New York: Doubleday, 1959

Kopp S. If you meet Buddha on the road, kill him! A modern pilgrimage through myth, legend, Zen and psychotherapy. London: Sheldon Press, 1972

Melia KM. Student nurses' accounts of their work and training: a qualitative analysis. Unpublished PhD Thesis. Edinburgh: University of Edinburgh, 1981

National Board for Nursing, Midwifery and Health Visiting for Scotland. Questioning of, or objecting to, participation in medical procedures. Edinburgh: SNB

Parsons T. On becoming a patient. In: Folta JR, Deck ES (eds). A sociological framework for patient care. Chichester: John Wiley, 1966

Raths L, Harmin M, Simon S. Values and teaching. Columbus, Ohio: Merrill 1966

Robinson D. The process of becoming ill. London: Routledge and Kegan Paul, 1971

Royal College of Nursing. Defining nursing. London: RCN, 2003

Rumbold G. Ethics in nursing practice. London: Baillière Tindall, 1986

Sampson C. The neglected ethic: religious and cultural factors in the care of patients. Maidenhead: McGraw-Hill, 1982

Simon S, Howe L, Kirschenbaum H. Values clarification. Revised ed. New York: A and W Visual Library, 1978

Stockwell F. The unpopular patient. London: RCN, 1972

Styles M. Nursing: towards a new endowment. St Louis: CV Mosby, 1983

Van Hooft S. Caring and ethics in nursing. In: Tschudin V (ed). Approaches to ethics: nursing beyond boundaries. Oxford: Elsevier, 2003

World Health Professions. Declaration on cloning. Geneva: ICN, 2002

3 Consent to care

■ CONTENTS

Patients frequently complain: 'They don't tell you anything', or 'I didn't realise it would be like this'. Now it may be true that the patient or relative was not given the required information, because the healthcare professional with whom they were in contact made the assumption that they would automatically realise what was involved, or the professional may have thought that the information had been given but failed to ascertain the level of the patient's understanding.

The Nursing and Midwifery Council's Code of Professional Conduct (Appendix I) states:

All patients and clients have a right to receive information about their condition. You must be sensitive to their needs and respect the wishes of those that refuse or are unable to receive information about their condition. Information should be accurate, truthful and presented in such a way as to make it easily understood. You may need to seek legal or professional

> *advice, or seek guidance from your employer, in relation to the giving or withholding of consent. (Paragraph 3.1)*

Within this statement are many areas that need elaboration if their intent is to be fully realised.

First is the idea that the patient has a 'right' to knowledge. The question of the rights and responsibilities of the nurse and patient were discussed in Chapter 2. One of the perceived rights of the patient was to receive information and the corresponding duty of the nurse was to provide such information. The paternal approach that was held for decades was that the doctor or nurse knows best and the patient should be grateful for the care given and not ask questions. It is true that some professionals still feel threatened when their practise is called into account but the increasing use of tools such as clinical audit and clinical governance have encouraged a greater acceptance of the need for critical appraisal. Some patients may abdicate any involvement in their care and resist discussion and information but these are becoming fewer as public knowledge of medical matters increases, due to media exploration of topics that were previously taboo.

How, then, is the nurse to ensure that information given to the patient is not only accurate and truthful but also understood? The first requirement is that the nurse must understand the issues involved.

NURSE EDUCATION

Recent years have seen a major change in the way nurses are educated. The apprenticeship system, which held sway from the days of Florence Nightingale, has been replaced by an academic approach in which nurses are required to understand the theoretical basis for the care given. The 'why' of care has to be coupled with the 'how'. No longer is care given routinely, because 'it has always been done that way'; care is given because that is the way in which that specific individual's needs may be met, and care is based on sound evidence of effectiveness.

The problem is that clinical knowledge does not stand still, and therefore emphasis has been given to continual professional development. It is not enough for a nurse to graduate or obtain registration and then practise with that knowledge for the next 30 years. PREP (Post-Registration Education and Practice) requires evidence of updating of knowledge and skill. There is a moral obligation for the nurse to keep up to date with current knowledge and practice. Alfred North Whitehead (1932), the philosopher of science noted that 'knowledge keeps no better than fish!'

Many avenues are open to enable nurses to continue their education. Knowledge may be updated through personal study and reflection or through attendance on a course. Many institutions offer modular courses, which may be taken part-time, either by attendance at classes or by distance learning. These modules may be aggregated to enable the student to obtain a recognised qualification such as a degree. Other courses enable specific clinical skills to be developed and others assist with managerial skills. Whatever the type of course undertaken it will enable the student to maintain a spirit of enquiry and prevent the stagnation of knowledge.

Another way in which the nurse may continue to develop is through mentoring. While there has been considerable discussion as to the role of mentor (Atwood, 1979; Brown, 1984; Burnard, 1989, 1990; Donovan, 1990), there is agreement that a mentor is an experienced nurse, who can offer support in clinical settings and assist in the development of reflective practice. (Details regarding the activity of mentoring are discussed more fully in Chapter 6.)

PATIENT AUTONOMY

It is important to realise that patients have personal autonomy and therefore have the right to agree or disagree with any action or treatment that is proposed, even if refusal may result in harm or death of themselves or, in the case of pregnant women, their fetus. This may be very difficult for doctors and nurses to accept but this can only be varied by a court of law. Listening to the patient may reveal their reason for refusal. Refusal may be overcome by adequate explanation but not by applying undue pressure to conform.

Consent can only be given (or refused) by a person who is legally competent and this must be presumed unless otherwise assessed by a suitably qualified practitioner. Consent can be given in writing, orally or by co-operation of the patient; however it is wise to have the decision in writing so that there is no possibility of confusion. If a patient is legally incompetent to make an informed decision the nurse should try to find out if their wishes had been previously expressed in an advanced statement, for example in a 'living will'. If such a statement exists, it is relevant to the current situation, there is no evidence that they had changed their mind, and the statement was made when the patient was legally competent, then their wishes should be respected. When there is no evidence as to the patient's wishes the clinical staff may make the decision that they feel is in the patient's best interests.

When a patient is mentally ill and incapable of making an informed decision the relatives or people close to the patient, including the psychiatrist, should be involved in making the decision.

It is important to realise that no one has the right to give consent on behalf of a legally competent adult. However, when dealing with children, in some circumstances a person with parental responsibility may give consent depending on the age and understanding of the child. In England and Wales, the age of consent is 16, in Scotland it is 12 and in Northern Ireland it is 17.

It is preferable that the person performing a procedure is the one to obtain consent, but in practice, if this task falls to the nurse she should ascertain what the medical practitioner has told the patient and whether it has been understood.

Consent is not always concerned with the living but may involve asking agreement to perform a post-mortem or to allow organ donation to take place. The medical practitioner or a specially trained transplant co-ordinator should obtain such consent. However, in some situations the nurse has built up trust with the deceased's relatives and may be asked to help in the explanations and discussions. Again, it is important to be truthful and to ensure that the whole truth is told. In the 1990s much distress was caused to relatives of deceased children when it was discovered that organs had been removed at post-mortem and kept for research. The relatives had given consent for the post-mortem but had no idea that their child's body was not intact when it was returned for burial. It is likely that if they had been asked for permission to retain organs or tissue this would, in many cases, have been given, but rightly, outrage was felt at the way in which this was assumed.

Informing and explaining

Once the nurse is certain of her own understanding of the issues involved it becomes important that she breaks this knowledge down into a form that is appropriate for the specific patient. This is not always as easy as it may appear. Some highly intelligent people have little idea of the functioning of their own bodies; others are avid readers of medical articles in popular magazines and have preconceived ideas. Children may have very different notions of their bodies and how they work and individuals with learning difficulties may also have limited understanding. Often the best approach is not to start with an explanation but with a question. Ask the patient what they understand or expect to happen, and prompt if necessary with supplementary questions until a clear picture emerges of the patient's view. From that point, it should be possible to commence an explanation of their condition and treatment and the areas for which consent may be required. Sometimes a simple drawing or diagram may be helpful. Medical terminology may need to be translated into lay, easily understood language – however it is vital that the patient does not feel that the nurse is 'talking down' to them. When the nurse feels that the explanation has been understood, and before any document is signed, the patient should be asked to say what they now feel is the situation.

Sometimes, in the effort of trying to explain the situation without frightening the patient, there is a temptation to 'water down' what is to happen or to discount any possible side effects. The Code emphasises the importance of truthfulness. It is vital that an individual is in possession of all the facts before giving consent to treatment. This also applies to discussions with relatives – remembering, however, the patient's right to confidentiality.

There may be occasions when the patient is unable to give consent, either because of their medical condition (for example, they may be unconscious), because of mental illness which precludes understanding, or in the case of a young child. In an emergency, when treatment is essential to preserve life, the nurse or doctor may provide treatment or care without consent, providing it is in the best interest of the patient.

ADVANCED DIRECTIVE

In recent years it has become possible for an individual to make an Advanced Statement, often described as a Living Will, in which the person expresses their desires with regard to medical treatment. The statement may cover the type of treatment the person would find acceptable, particularly in the case of potentially terminal illness, and whether resuscitation should be carried out. Although the legal status of such a document is ambiguous most healthcare professionals would abide by its provisions. It is more difficult to deal a situation in which such wishes become known at a later stage when treatment has already been initiated. Particularly difficult are requests to discontinue treatment, including shutting down life support machines.

The Department of Health for England has an advisory group dealing with good practice in consent and this group is attempting to deal with such matters in detail.

RESEARCH

When involving people in research studies it is important that each patient or subject is fully informed as to the purpose of the trial, any possible dangers and the fact that it may not directly be of benefit to them before they are asked for consent. Double blind trials, where neither the researcher nor the subject knows what treatment (usually drugs) the subject is receiving, need special vigilance, particularly if unforeseen and potentially dangerous side effects occur. Recent years have seen trials stopped before completion because of such ill effects or because the benefit of one approach is obviously superior to another. It is obviously immoral to continue to put a patient at risk, even if extra knowledge regarding the treatment would be valuable for others.

The Code emphasises the importance of truth and the absence of any form of deception. All actions relating to patients or clients must be for their benefit in the long run. Some treatments, such as chemotherapy for cancer, may seem in the immediate future to be anything but beneficial but the patient must understand this and the intended eventual benefit prior to giving consent. Benjamin and Curtis (1981, p.62) say that 'deception is a form of manipulation, like coercion and rational persuasion; it is a way of inducing others to do what one wants them to do'. Tschudin (2003) argues that 'deception corrodes trust by making light of truth, and that in turn is destructive to helping and caring relationships'.

■ QUESTIONS FOR REFLECTION AND DISCUSSION

1 Can you envisage any situation where you may act without obtaining informed consent?

2 How can the healthcare professional ensure that their knowledge is up to date?

REFERENCES

Atwood AH. The mentor in clinical practice. Nursing Outlook 1979; 27: 714-771

Benjamin M, Curtis J. Ethics in nursing. New York: Oxford University Press, 1981

Brown BJ. The dean as mentor. Nursing Health Care 1984; 5(2): 88-91

Burnard P. The role of mentor. Journal of District Nursing1989; 8(3): 8-10

Burnard P. Is anyone here a mentor? Nursing Standard 1990; 4: 37-46

Department of Health Advisory Group on Consent. Discussion document. London: HMSO

Donovan J. The concept and role of the mentor. Nursing Education Today 1990; 10: 294-298

Tschudin V. Ethics in nursing: the caring relationship. 3rd ed. London: Elsevier, 2003

UKCC. PREP: Post-registration education and practice. London: UKCC

Whitehead AN. The aims of education. London: Benn, 1932

4 Working Together

The explosion of knowledge that occurred in the 20th century has made it impossible for one person to possess all the knowledge and skill that is required to treat and care for the sick in society. This has resulted in the emergence of a variety of professional groups; some of them, such as physiotherapy and radiography, evolving from tasks at one time included in nursing. In addition within these professional groups, including nursing, specialisation has occurred. While this has allowed highly qualified and skilled practitioners to deal with specific aspects of patient treatment and care, it has also meant that teams of people have had to come together to ensure that all aspects of care are adequately covered.

WORKING AS A TEAM

Working as a member of a team is therefore a common experience for all today's health professionals, and one with which nurses are very familiar. A typical ward team comprises a ward manager (ward sister or charge nurse), other registered nurses (staff nurses and clinical nurse specialists), nurses who are learners, physiotherapists and possibly physiotherapy students, a social worker, and maybe others depending on the nature of the ward or unit. There will also be medical staff: consultant physicians or surgeons, registrars, house officers, and medical students attached to the consultant's 'firm'. In addition there will be healthcare assistants, a ward clerk, ward receptionist, domestic staff, and in some cases a porter. A formidable array of people, all there ostensibly to 'care' for the patient. However, this apparently common goal may not be perceived, in the short term, with the same level of importance by all members of the team. The medical consultant may be concerned to show efficiency by having high bed occupancy and a rapid patient turnover in order to reduce his list of patients waiting admission. The domestic may want to have the most highly polished floors in the hospital; the nursing student may want the opportunity to carry out new techniques; the medical student may be preoccupied with the study of interesting cases and the registrar anxious to complete a piece of research. None of these aims are intrinsically bad, providing that the needs of the patients remain paramount, and this can be achieved with good leadership.

Who is the leader? This remains a contentious question. The medical consultant may consider that as it is normally a clinical decision to admit or discharge patients, the team leader should be a doctor. The ward manager has to co-ordinate the activities of most of the team and the administration of care, and this may be considered the leadership role. For a patient whose main goal is to learn to walk again and regain independence the physiotherapist may seem to be the key person. Obviously all members of the team are important and the fact that emphasis may shift during the stay of the patient makes co-operative working vital.

It is essential that each individual recognises the contribution made by the others involved in the care of patients so that the most appropriate skills are utilised. Competition is not the best way to ensure that the goals of patient cure and care are realised. Section 4 of the Code states: 'As a registered nurse or midwife you must co-operate with others in the team.'

Although first thoughts assume that this refers to fellow professionals, the Code goes on to emphasise: 'The team includes the patient or client, the patient's or client's family, informal carers, and health and social care professionals in the National Health Service, independent and voluntary sectors.' (Section 4.1)

It is sometimes difficult to recognise the position of the patient or client as part of the team, even though without them there would be no need for a team. The government of the UK has recently set up a Commission for Patient and Public Involvement in Health (2002). The Minister of Health is reported as saying:

> The NHS belongs to the public. They have a right to be fully involved and consulted about how local NHS services are planned, delivered and how they can be best improved. (The Times 2nd January 2003)

It will be interesting to see if this involvement spreads to clinical areas.

The question may be raised as to whether all team members are of equal worth. The answer raises another question: in what sense 'equal'? Obviously not all have the same knowledge and skill; some will have different attitudes and as already discussed individual goals may vary. Nevertheless, if all are needed for the effective care of the patient, then all should be equally valued for their contribution. Section 4.2 of the Code states: 'You are expected to work co-operatively within teams and to respect the skills, expertise and contributions of your colleagues. You must treat them fairly and without discrimination.' The apostle Paul expresses this most succinctly when considering the part played by church members in Corinth. He compares the church to the human body in which each part is different yet all are essential to the full and effective functioning of the person: 'if all were one part, where would the body be?' As it is, there are many parts but one body. The eye cannot say to the hand: 'I don't need you'. And the head cannot say to the feet: 'I don't need you'. On the contrary, those parts of the body that seem to be weaker are nonetheless indispensable – so there should be no division in the body, but its parts should have equal concern for each other. All are needed for a smooth running and effective caring unit.

The medical profession

The doctor has often been accorded supremacy within the team due to the fact that as already discussed, it is often a medical prerogative to admit and discharge patients. However, there are other factors which may tend to ensure that the doctor is seen as more important than other team members. One important factor is that, until recently, the doctor was the only person in the team to have benefited from higher education and hence other team members felt unable to challenge his or her views on the way the patient was perceived. This is no longer the case: most professional groups are now educated to degree level and many specialist practitioners in subjects allied to medicine not only have first degrees but doctorates. This has given them the confidence to question medical decisions. At one time doctors were traditionally male and nurses female and that, coupled with the fact that doctors were frequently of higher social class than nurses, enhanced their status. The increase in female doctors and male nurses has helped to change attitudes so that each member of the team is more likely to be accorded the respect and recognition they earn rather than to have their status ascribed to them merely by virtue of the role they fill.

EXTENDED ROLES OF THE NURSE

In the past decade nurses have taken on a variety of functions, many of which were previously the province of the doctor. One such role relates to the provision of a call centre, NHS Direct, that provides advice on medical matters to anyone who phones in. The nurses who operate these centres work to protocols which allow them to advise on most common problems. If in doubt, the caller is advised to seek medical help straight away. Although most doctors, especially general practitioners, opposed this service, callers appreciate the system and feel reassured by the advice given. There is no evidence that patient safety has been compromised and the original hostility to the service is abating.

Other roles where the nurse has become the first point of contact for a person seeking help are those of nurse practitioners in health centres, and triage nurses in accident and emergency departments. Nurses also run specialist clinics for patients with asthma, diabetes and other chronic conditions, while others specialise in giving support to patients with a stoma, following heart surgery and so on. Nurses are now beginning to perform some routine surgical procedures and other tasks formerly carried out by junior hospital doctors. While the shortage of doctors has given the impetus to these developments there is little doubt that nurses are capable of filling these roles.

These changes have helped to break down some of the barriers between medicine and nursing but have also meant that more traditional nursing tasks are now carried out by unregistered staff such as health care assistants.

Learning together

Attempts are being made to allow members of the varying healthcare professional groups to share at least some aspects of their education. In a document published in 2001 the UKCC recorded institutions where this practice was occurring and recommended that it be increased. If professionals learn together it is likely that they will gain a more accurate understanding of each other's roles, and co-operation in practice may be enhanced.

Conscientious objection

Occasionally conflict may arise between team members, usually due to each person holding different goals, or values regarding patient care. Sometimes these differences relate to fundamental issues such as the practice of euthanasia, abortion or genetic engineering. In these cases full and frank discussion is needed between all members of the team, including the patient. Where agreement cannot be reached, and the law does not provide guidance, provision must be made for conscientious objection so certain members of the team may withdraw from the situation. Although accountability to the team, including the patient, is important, the individual also has the right to be accountable to him/herself so that they can 'live with' themselves. The right to make a stand on a matter of conscience should be possible without organisational or professional backlash. To ensure the safety of the patient it is important that possible contentious views are aired in advance of a specific situation arising so that withdrawal is anticipated and appropriate action taken.

Whistle blowing

Sometimes the behaviour of one or more members of a team may give rise to concern, not only over a specific situation, but also with regard to general practice. In such a situation any individual who feels this concern should not hesitate to raise the matter with a higher authority. This is easier said than done – there are many instances in the past where individuals who have taken this step have been both ignored and victimised. A high profile case in Bristol (UK) has brought this type of situation to the attention of all health professional groups and, even more importantly, to the attention of the general public. In this case, the main complainant was an anaesthetist who was concerned about the health of children undergoing major cardiac surgery, which was associated with a high death rate. Although he complained to the surgeons concerned, to hospital management and to the local and national health authorities, his view was overridden and eventually he left the country to work elsewhere. Finally, as a result of other professional complaints and concerns made public by relatives, the matter was investigated. One surgeon was struck off the medical register, another had a limit placed on his practice and an administrator, who was also a doctor, had his medical registration revoked. This latter case emphasises that although, as a manager, he was not working as a doctor at the time, this individual's medical knowledge should have made him aware of the seriousness of the allegations. Once an individual is a registered as a professional, in any discipline, they are always a professional, and accountable for professional practice. A public enquiry made recommendations to prevent such a situation recurring; however, no amount of recommendation can substitute for personal integrity and accountability.

There may be occasions when the performance of a team member may give rise to concern because of physical inability. This can be in the form of illness, which the team member is trying to hide, and in some cases it may be due to abuse of drugs or alcohol or to stress. Sympathy for the individual often results in other team members covering up for the sick colleague by trying to do their work and by checking their performance. Although this may appear to be a kindness, in reality it merely exacerbates the problem. The team member needs treatment and the safety of patients or clients must not be compromised.

In the Code, Section 4.5: 'When working as a member of a team, you remain accountable for your professional conduct, any care you provide, and any omission on your part.' Section 4.7 states: 'You have a duty to co-operate with any internal or external investigations.' The safety of patients is paramount and there is no place for misplaced loyalty.

Nurses who find themselves in a situation where attempts to change inappropriate or dangerous practice are frustrated, despite having taken all the correct steps to bring the matter to conclusion, and/or find themselves victimised because of the action taken, may receive help and backing from the Royal College of Nursing.

The Public Interest Disclosure Act (1998) which came into effect in 1999 should help workers who are victimised or sacked for whistle blowing by providing support and compensation for dismissal, loss of earnings and/or distress. To date there is little evidence that this has occurred.

What is clear is that accurate records are required if any headway is to be made.

Records

One of the essential tools of any effective teamwork is clear unambiguous communication. This may be face to face but frequently has to take place via records. In the Code, Section 4.4 spells this out clearly:

> *Health care records are a tool of communication within the team. You must ensure that the records of the patient or client are an accurate account of treatment, care planning and delivery. It should be consecutive, written with the involvement of the patient or client wherever practicable and completed as soon as possible after the event has occurred. It should provide clear evidence of the care planned, the decisions made, the care delivered and the information shared.*

The question as to who should have access to these records is discussed in the chapter on confidentiality, but it is important to recognise the patient's right to have access. If the records are kept electronically then this is covered by the Data Protection Act (1984), which states: 'Individuals about whom data is held (data subjects) have a right to be informed about its nature and contents.' This statement also highlights another important point, that the patient is a member of the team.

Patient as team member

The days of 'the doctor knows best', or 'keep the patient in the dark' have almost gone. The public is now better educated than ever before regarding their body, possible disease processes and available treatments. This is due to the rapid rise in medical articles in the popular press and on television. Sometimes such media representation may portray an exaggerated picture and by its dramatic representation either induce unnecessary anxiety or raise false hopes. Nevertheless, most members of the public now expect to be kept unformed as to their healthcare status and the options available for treatment and care. By including the patient as a team member it is likely that better decisions will be made and co-operation achieved.

■ QUESTIONS FOR REFLECTION AND DISCUSSION

1 What are the benefits and shortcomings of working in a team?

2 What would you do if you felt that a patient's rights were being compromised?

REFERENCES

Apostle Paul.1 Corinthians Chap.12: 19-23 Holy Bible. New International Version

Data Protection Act. London: HMSO, 1984

Ministry of Health. Inquiry into Bristol Royal Infirmary. London: HMSO, 2000

Public Interest Disclosure Act. London: HMSO, 1998

UKCC. Fitness for practice and purpose: the report of the UKCC's post-commission development group. London: UKCC, 2001

5 Confidentiality

Clause 5 of the Code states: 'As a registered nurse or midwife you must protect confidential information.' Such a statement may appear self-evident but there are many situations when it may be challenged.

The need for confidentiality is one that was recognised as far back as the days of the Hippocratic Oath, which stated:

> *Whatsoever things I see or hear concerning the life of men, in my attendance on the sick or even apart therefrom, which ought not to be noised abroad, I will keep silence thereon, counting such things as sacred secrets.*

Today newly qualified doctors at graduation, and indeed some nurses, are expected to endorse the content, if not the exact words, of the original statement. Whether actual words are spoken in the form of an oath or not, all healthcare workers are expected to adhere to the same principles.

Table 5.1 The pattern of doctor/nurse–patient relationship

| Doctor/Nurse | | Patient/Client | |
Right	Duty	Right	Duty
Information	Confidentiality	Knowledge	Reveal data
Access to data	Treatment	Confidentiality	Cooperation

The important concept here is that of 'trust'. Without it, no therapeutic relationship can develop or be sustained between healthcare worker and patient or client. The level of trust placed by the patient or client in the doctor or nurse is very high indeed. It results in the disclosure of personal details, the submission to intimate examination (both physical and mental), and the agreement to, and co-operation in, often unpleasant treatment and regimens. In return for this trust, the patient has the right to expect that information given and details of mind and body revealed would be respected and only used in a therapeutic manner for the purpose for which it was given (Section 5.1).

RIGHTS AND DUTIES

This is another interesting example of rights and duties being, in effect, opposite sides of the same coin (see Table 5.1).

By agreeing to enter into a relationship with a healthcare professional the patient tacitly agrees to divulge personal information. However, one of the problems is that the patient is rarely cared for by one individual, but by a team made up of a variety of workers. In this situation it is vital that all team members have access to relevant information. Generally patients are aware of this and therefore their consent to the sharing of this information is implied (Section 5.1).

One problem is to decide which individuals are team members and therefore who should have access to the records. It may be clearly understood by the patient that the doctor and nurse need information and probably few would question the need for the physiotherapist to have access to the patient's file, but has the hospital chaplain the same right of access? What about the wide range of students who may be involved in the organisation? In certain cases it may be necessary for specific consent to be obtained to widen the right of access.

The patient may regard some information as of such a sensitive nature that a request is made that access to it be restricted. This request should be honoured and if it is subsequently found that an individual not originally considered to need the information now requires it for the patient's good, then specific consent must be obtained. This can cause difficulties when a patient confides in a nurse and requests that no other person be told, yet the nurse recognises that this information is needed by the doctor if appropriate treatment is to take place. In this case the nurse should not divulge the information but explain to the patient why the doctor needs to be told.

The nurse may acquire other information, which the patient expects to be kept confidential, such as their infection with HIV or even in some cases involvement with drug dealing or other criminal activity. Such information places the nurse in a difficult position, as the trust of the specific patient has to be balanced against the good of the community. Section 5.3 of the Code deals with this problem and states: 'If a patient or client withholds consent, or if consent cannot be obtained, for whatever reason, disclosures may be made only when they can be justified in the public interest (usually where disclosure is essential to protect the patient or client or someone else from significant harm) or they are required by a court of law.' Section 5.4 states: 'Where there is an issue of child protection, you must act at all times in accordance with national and local policies.'

There are, therefore, some rare occasions when the rights of the individual have to be surrendered in order to achieve a greater good. The nurse may sometimes have difficulty in deciding when the good of society requires such action. Should the fact that a patient is found to have been trafficking in dangerous drugs be disclosed? There is no easy answer to such questions. The individual nurse should seek advice from superiors, other professionals and also their professional organisation. The implication of disclosure must be considered from all angles before a decision is made.

While the discussion so far has focused on professional healthcare workers, there are others, such as medical secretaries and record clerks, who also handle the patient documents. They also are bound by their work contract of employment to maintain confidentiality. Some Trusts have found this discretion regarding the sharing of information difficult to deal with and have refused to allow some team members, such as the hospital chaplain, access to notes. There may be occasions when the material is so sensitive that this action is appropriate but individual access should be considered on a 'need to know' basis and not by a blanket embargo.

The Department of Health and Social Security set up a working group on confidentiality, which suggested the following wording to be included in contracts for staff other than healthcare professionals:

> *In the course of your duties you may have access to confidential material about patients, members of staff or other healthcare service business. On no account must information relating to*

identifiable patients be divulged to anyone other than authorised persons, for example medical, nursing or other professional staff, as appropriate, who are concerned directly with care, diagnosis and/or treatment of the patient. If you are in any doubt whatsoever as to the authority of a person or body asking for information of this nature you must seek advice from your superior officer. Similarly, no information of a personal or confidential nature concerning individual members of staff should be divulged to anyone without the proper authority having first been given. Failure to observe these rules will be regarded by your employers as a serious misconduct which could result in serious disciplinary action being taken against you, including dismissal. (DHSS, 1985)

The fact that confidential information is held in patients' records has been a contentious issue. Patients have been suspicious of what has been recorded, especially as for many years they were not allowed access to their own notes. This is no longer the situation although in many areas patients have to actively seek access to their records before they are made available.

The Data Protection Act (1984) legally protects 'automatically processed information' which normally means computerised records. Under this Act any material kept on a computer record for 40 days or over must be available for inspection. Data users, that is the individuals who control the contents and use of personal data which is automatically processed, must register the type of data they hold, how it is obtained and the purpose for which it is required.

Relatives

There may be occasions when relatives of the patient or client seek information about their condition, treatment and prognosis. Section 5.2 of the Code states: 'You should seek patients' and clients' wishes regarding the sharing of information with their family and others.' The use of the phrase 'next of kin' is fraught with difficulty in that there are now many stable partnerships, both heterosexual and homosexual, to which conventional kinship may not apply. In such cases, and when family members feel that they have a right to know what is happening to their relative, it is vital that the patient's wishes are sought and followed. If the patient or client is unable to express their wishes or give permission the nurse should seek advice from colleagues and follow local policies.

Telling the truth

Patients, quite rightly, ask questions regarding their illness and prognosis. Perhaps the question most dreaded by any nurse, but especially by the student on night duty is: 'Am I going to die, nurse?'

Breaking bad news is something that all healthcare professionals have to do at some time or other and it is important that the fact is faced before a difficult situation arises. The immediate response to such a question is, in some way or other, to be reassuring. An evasive reply ('We are all going to die one day') or a direct lie, are not appropriate responses. However, how the truth is told and who should tell the truth varies. It is often useful to find out why the patient is asking the question. Many patients actually know the answer but want to raise the subject so that other concerns such as pain relief, telling relatives, or making a will can be dealt with. Sometimes the nurse may genuinely not know the answer but will have to refer the matter to the senior nurse or doctor. Whatever happens, the patient must have a reply that they understand and that is truthful. To do this the nurse needs knowledge, skill, intuition and empathy.

However, the nurse is not alone in this situation but is part of a team, and the team should have guidelines as to how such a situation is met. Some doctors have excellent communication skills and prefer to be the person to explain to the patient their prognosis; others feel that this is best carried out by the nurse. Either way, whatever the news, it must be backed with reassurance regarding the care that will be provided. It is essential that the patient is given time to ask questions and that opportunity is given for further talks. This is so that at all times the patient realises that not only is the truth being told, but that the staff really care and will do all that is possible to ensure their wellbeing and comfort.

Another difficult situation may develop when patients wish to withhold information from relatives, and visa versa. This can be regarding diagnosis, treatment, prognosis or issues such as whether to resuscitate. While the concern of relatives is understandable the patient's confidentiality is the nurse's prime concern and relatives may have to be gently told that the patient does not want information given.

Under English law, relatives do not have power to make decisions regarding medical treatment of a family member, nor can they insist on treatment or non-treatment. The issue of resuscitation (and whether not to resuscitate) is the final responsibility of the doctor. However, all members of the healthcare team need to be comfortable with the decision and if the patient is mentally competent it should be discussed with him prior to an order being made.

The days of health professionals adopting a paternal approach to patients are over. Patients require and deserve honesty.

■ **QUESTIONS FOR REFLECTION AND DISCUSSION**

1 Under what circumstances might you break confidentiality?

2 Are there any situations when you might feel it inappropriate to tell a patient the truth?

REFERENCES

Data Protection Act. London: HMSO, 1984

Department of Health and Social Security. Report of the confidentiality working group of the DHSS steering group on health service information. London: DHSS, 1985

Nursing and Midwives Council. Code of Professional Conduct. London: NMC, 2002

6 Competence

It may seem obvious that a registered nurse or midwife needs to maintain their professional knowledge and competence, but this is the substance of Paragraph 6 of the Code. Indeed, lack of competence is a threat to patient safety (other aspects are dealt with in Chapter 8). At its inception the Nursing and Midwifery Council (NMC) was given the power to remove from the register nurses or midwives who were demonstrated to be incompetent. This power was not used immediately due to difficulties with the definition of 'incompetence'; however, in January 2003 the NMC issued the following definition of incompetence:

> *A lack of knowledge, skill or judgement which may be accompanied by a negative attitude. This is of such a nature or extent that the nurse, midwife or heath visitor is unfit to practice, and that such concerns having been drawn to the attention of the practitioner, he or she has undergone training*

*and supervision but has failed to make the required
improvement to practice, or has refused to undergo further
training or supervision.*

The NMC has notified the professions that, from November 2003, it intends to take action on practitioners who are shown to be incompetent.

KNOWLEDGE AND SKILL

Paragraph 6.1 of the Code states: 'You must keep your knowledge and skills up-to-date throughout your working life. In particular you should take part regularly in learning activities that develop your competence and performance.' The need for appropriate knowledge and skill has already been emphasised in preceding chapters as without it the patient cannot be kept informed or safe; this is the bedrock of professional practice.

The importance of maintaining up-to-date knowledge and the need for life-long learning was recognised by the fore-runner of the Nursing and Midwifery Council, the UKCC. In 1995 it published a document entitled *Post-Registration Education and Practice* (UKCC, 1995). This requires all nurses to demonstrate that, in a three-year period prior to the renewal of registration, they have undergone five days or 35 hours of learning activity relevant to their work in order to maintain their registration. This does not have to be in the form of attendance at lectures or a specific course but can include any activity which can be shown to increase the nurse's knowledge. In addition nurses have to keep a personal professional portfolio indicating their continuing professional development. This professional learning development will normally occur during their clinical practice. These recommendations came into force from April 2001, and the UKCC had the right to audit these practices. Interesting all the publications from the UKCC regarding these developments have the aims of the body on the title page: 'Protecting the public through professional standards'.

Personal development of this type is required for a nurse to be held accountable for the care given.

ACCOUNTABILITY

Nurses are frequently reminded that they are responsible for their actions but they may not always be held accountable. It is necessary for the nurse not only to understand the reasons for the care and treatment given but also to understand the anticipated outcome. For example, a nurse may be responsible for getting a patient out of bed 12 hours after major surgery; however, to be held accountable for this action the nurse must understand the reason and possible outcomes for it. This means that the 'accountable' nurse will understand the dangers of immobility, the risk of deep vein thrombosis and also the possible unacceptable fall in blood pressure that may occur, thus increasing the risk of shock. Understanding all these factors, the nurse will be able to make a decision regarding the action to be taken for that specific patient, which may not be the same decision as would be taken for the patient in the next bed.

It is quite clear therefore that to be accountable demands knowledge so that the relative benefits, or otherwise, of alternative forms of action may be assessed. This means that while a student may be responsible for care given to a patient, as a learner it may not be appropriate to expect accountability as the necessary knowledge or skill may not yet have been acquired. Accountability also requires authority to be able to make alternative decisions, and this cannot be held by a learner.

To summarise, to be accountable the nurse requires not only appropriate up-to-date knowledge and skills, but also permission to act with a reasonable degree of autonomy.

Much of this development occurs during practical care-giving and this may be assisted by the use of a mentor; that is, an experienced nurse who can guide and help the learner develop a critical, self-reflective attitude to care given.

THE MENTOR RELATIONSHIP

Darling (1984) found in her research that there were three 'absolute requirements for a significant mentoring relationship'. These were attraction, action and affect.

Attraction

It is deemed vital that both people like and respect each other. Arguably, as the relationship develops, a transference relationship will evolve (Burton, 1977). The term transference is usually reserved as a descriptor of the nature of the relationship which develops between a psychotherapist and her client. It signifies that the client comes to see the therapist as having personal characteristics (usually positive ones) that are reminiscent of the client's parents. All this normally takes place at a pre- or unconscious level so the client does not readily see that it is happening. The net result is usually that the client 'idealises' the therapist and becomes very dependent on her. One of the aims of therapy is to help the client to resolve this transference relationship and thus live a less dependent and more independent life (Burnard, 1989). It seems likely that the relationship between the student and the mentor is also likely to involve transference, particularly as the mentor is already cast in the role of 'expert'. All this suggests that the mentor should be chosen very carefully. Who should do the choosing is a matter for debate.

It is possible that the 'attraction' could also include emotional and sexual attraction. The ethical position is clear – at least in theory. The relationship between mentor and student should remain 'platonic', given the tacit contract that exists between teachers, clinical staff and students. Life is rarely as simple as that, however, and the issue of how to cope with more involved relationships needs to be recognised and addressed.

Action

In terms of the 'action' role of the mentor, the student is likely to want to use the mentor as a role model. Again, by definition, the mentor is seen as an expert: someone who has achieved the various skills that are deemed necessary for effective practice and who is able to use and pass on these skills. In a sense, this aspect of mentoring may be equivalent to the 'sitting with Nellie' approach that some forms of apprenticeship training employ. 'Sitting with Nellie' refers to the idea that by watching a skilled person those skills will be learnt. Traditionally there has been an element of this approach in the past training of students. Just being with a qualified person was sometimes seen as enough to encourage students to learn and develop skills. Whether or not this was ever the case is another debatable point! A certain skill in coaching seems to be a requirement of a mentor. The ability to break down skills into their component parts and to teach them, and then the ability to demonstrate their use with the appropriate accompanying effect, is another skill to aim for.

Affect

From the 'affective' point of view, the mentor needs to be able to act in a supportive role. She should be able to encourage the student, enhance her self-confidence and teach her to be constructively critical of what she sees and does. This critical appraisal of nursing actions will result in a 'reflective practitioner'; one who constantly endeavours 'to do better next time'. Again, this aspect of mentoring may re-open the debate about the likelihood of transference occurring. If transference does occur it is important that the mentor is able to deal with it. The mentor must also be able to close the relationship and know how to say 'goodbye'. This may not be easy because of the possible 'counter-transference' that may have occurred due to the mentor's feelings for the student. At best, however, the mentoring relationship will mirror the truly therapeutic relationship that the student will be able to use as a pattern for relationships with patients.

If such a relationship develops and is sustained, it is likely to be very valuable for the student and, no doubt, for the mentor. On the other hand there are potential problems because the student is, by nature of the relationship, in an inferior relationship with the mentor who, of necessity, is the dominant figure. It is not, and cannot be, a relationship of equals. Most writing on adult education suggests that it should be a matter of negotiation between teacher and learner, and be an exercise in shared learning and meeting the student's own perceived needs (Brookfield, 1987). The adult, so this argument goes, needs to use what he learns as he learns it; he needs to be treated as an equal in a partnership that leads along a road of inquiry; he needs to have his self-concept protected as he goes. Whether such demands for negotiation and equality can be met within the constraints of a mentor-student relationship is unclear. It seems more likely that the mentor will be seen as a benign (or not so benign) father or mother substitute. Some may find such a portrayal over-dramatic, but as we have noted, the perfectly respectable notion of transference depends on the unconscious designation of the other person as a surrogate parent.

There is also the problem of the mentor's own development. There is nothing worse than a 'guru' who feels that she has gained enlightenment and that all she needs to do is to sit back and pass on pearls of wisdom. The requirements of PREP would prevent this happening as it relates to all registered nurses.

As already stated, the Code (Sections 6.2 and 6.3) stresses not only the need for knowledge and skill, but also an ability to practice competently without supervision, and for the insight to recognise when knowledge and skills are lacking and therefore practice may be dangerous to the patient. The acknowledgement of personal shortcomings is difficult, particularly when there is a shortage of staff, but if the patient is to receive safe care it must be accepted and a request made for supervision until competence is gained.

To appreciate the limits of one's competence it is necessary to develop self-awareness. What is self-awareness and how can it be developed? To answer these questions it may be helpful to investigate the concept of 'self'. This is a difficult concept much debated by philosophers, theologians, psychologists and sociologists and there are many ways of approaching it (Williams, 1973; Canfield & Wells, 1976; Rogers, 1951;

Macquarie, 1973). All have made a useful contribution to the debate and the analysis used here is only one way of approaching the subject.

Following the work of Carl Jung, five aspects of self may be identified: sensing, thinking, feeling, intuiting, and body experience. The first four of these aspects Jung summarises:

> *The essential function of sensation is to establish that something exists, thinking tells us what it means, feeling what its value is and intuition summarises whence it comes and whither it goes. (Jung 1983 p. 144)*

Sensing

The first aspect is sensation. It might be said that everything that is thought about or felt is experienced first through one of the five special senses: hearing, seeing, tasting, smelling and touching, of which the first two are the most highly developed.

It is easy, however, for attention to the senses to be lost. Very often a person is so distracted by their thoughts and feelings that they fail to pay attention to what they feel or hear. In this way the person fails to take full advantage of an educational encounter; or alternatively a considerable amount of the patient's communication is lost. In order to appreciate fully the inputs that are being received through the senses, a person must concentrate on them. A simple experiment may serve to drive this point home. Stop reading this book for a moment and pay close attention to what you can hear around you. As you do so, you will suddenly realise how much auditory input has been filtered out prior to undertaking the experiment.

Such filtering is essential at times, but at others it is necessary to resist the shutting out process and pay close attention to what is going on around you. Part of becoming self-aware is the process of 'noticing': simply paying attention to what is being seen and heard. The development of such attention can help increase the accuracy of reporting, improve observational skills and increase resistance to making snap judgements and evaluations. The person who is paying conscious attention to what they are seeing or hearing gathers accurate data and is therefore in a better position to make considered judgements. Such a position is in line with the Code's requirement that nurses acknowledge their limitations of competence.

Thinking

Once information enters in through one of the senses, it is thought about. Thinking, here, refers to the process of puzzling, pondering, analysing and criticising. It is essential that the person reflects upon what they know, on whether or not what they know is accurate and what they need to develop in terms of knowledge. In this sense, it is necessary to develop a continuous and consistent ability to be critical: to question regularly what is held to be true. This is not a comfortable process! It is sometimes easier to hang on to an old set of beliefs that have been useful in the past than to question the validity of those beliefs. It is far less comfortable still to adopt Marx's favourite maxim, 'doubt everything' (Singer, 1980).

This inner reflection on knowledge and upon its validity and present day utility value is again part of the Code's requirements. To acknowledge limitations and to refuse to accept certain delegated functions is to first have pondered upon one's own knowledge and skills base.

Feelings

This term refers to the whole spectrum of emotions that may be felt, ranging on the one hand from elation, to, on the other hand, profound depression. What is important is that the individual develops the ability to identify and acknowledge her feelings in any given situation. In nursing it is often easier (and sometimes encouraged) either to ignore or rationalise feelings as they occur in day-to-day practice and even to pretend that they do not exist. This is evident in the popular image of the nurse as an implacable, objective carer, who has somehow learned to detach herself from the issue of emotion. Quite how this image has arisen is unclear but its effects are well documented. Bond (1986) points out that consistent bottling up of emotion can lead to frustration, anxiety and burnout.

Nurses have a reputation for 'coping' and this is seen as a positive attribute. Unfortunately it may result in individuals being placed in situations where it is not possible for them to 'cope'. Some of these situations are obvious; for example, the student who is asked to carry out a task that she has not yet been taught. Other situations are more complex. Sometimes the lack of competence is not due to lack of knowledge or skill, but due to stress. One of the results of continuous work overload may be burnout (Shubin, 1978; Storlie, 1979). This may be defined as an evolutionary and insidious process of emotional exhaustion occurring as a consequence of being exposed to chronic job-related stress factors. Three degrees of burnout may be identified. Characteristics of the first degree include short-lived bouts of irritability, fatigue, worry and a tendency perpetually to view work situations and colleagues in a pessimistic and negative manner. Second-degree burnout may be viewed as a worsening of the situation, accompanied by feelings of failure, lack of interest in work and a sense of powerlessness and inadequacy. With the onset of the third degree comes the development of psychosomatic ailments, excessive sick leave, the over-use of alcohol and perhaps the excessive use of tranquillisers. With all these changes comes a deep sense of dissatisfaction. This is often marked by a sarcastic and cynical manner and a tendency to be judgmental and over-critical of others. Such attitudes may result in a failure to co-operate in team working and to lead to incompetence.

The individual may not have insight into the situation into which they are falling and this is a case where the care of a colleague needs to be demonstrated. It is tempting to take the easy way out by covering for the person by completing their tasks. This may ensure the immediate safety of the patient, but it is only a short-term solution. A variety of factors may contribute to the development of burnout. Age and health are important physical factors; personal relationships, home life and other social factors all play a part. Psychological factors such as the personality of the individual and their problem-solving skills influence the degree to which nurses avoid or develop burnout. Ideological factors, such as how authentic the individual feels in her role, the degree to which she feels fulfilled in her job, and how much she is able to invest in relationships with patients and others all play a part in coping with, or avoiding, burnout. Organisational factors such as career position and future prospects need to be taken into account, too.

RESPONSIBILITY FOR OTHERS

While the individual nurse is personally responsible for her competence and actions this does not absolve colleagues from taking action. Altruism should not be reserved for patients but should be available to colleagues. Part of this caring relates to the way in which work is allocated. When delegating work it is important to ensure that the individual both understands the task and is capable of carrying it out. This is particularly important when dealing with learners but applies to all aspects of delegation. Section 6.4 of the Code states: 'You have a duty to facilitate students of nursing and midwifery and others to develop their competence.'

RESEARCH

One way in which an individual can maintain their level of knowledge and be certain of carrying out care with the best level of up-to-date knowledge, is by participating in and applying validated research (Section 6.5).

In the past twenty years, research into nursing practice has gradually been accumulating. However it is true to say that much of it is unknown to the nurse at the bedside. Some of the blame for this situation lies with the researchers who, in order to advance their academic credibility, only publish their findings in academic journals which are not read by the majority of nurses. Some blame must also be attached to the Research Assessment Exercise whereby universities score points (and then attract funding) according to the level of academic research produced. Unfortunately, even when research is published in a readily accessible format, there is often resistance to implementing the findings. Some of this resistance is due to inertia; change takes time and energy and it is easier to maintain the old practices. If the benefits of change have been clearly demonstrated by the research and the nurse acknowledges that fact, then failure to implement the recommendations is clearly a breech of Clause 6.5 of the Code, which states: 'You have a responsibility to deliver care based on current evidence, best practice and where applicable, validated research when it is available.'

In nursing, as in law, 'ignorance is no defence' so the need to keep up to date is essential if the nurse is not to be accused of professional misconduct.

■ QUESTIONS FOR REFLECTION AND DISCUSSION

1 What is a reflective practitioner?

2 How are you keeping your knowledge and skills up to date?

3 How can you avoid suffering burnout?

REFERENCES

Bond M. Stress and self-awareness: a guide for nurses. London: Heinemann, 1986

Brookfield SD. Developing critical thinkers: challenging adults to explore alternative ways of thinking and acting. Milton Keynes: Open University Press, 1987

Burnard P. The role of the mentor. Journal of District Nursing 1989; 8(3): 8-10

Burton A. The mentoring dynamic in the therapeutic transformation. The American Journal of Psychoanalysis 1977; 37: 115-122

Canfield J, Wells HC. 100 ways to enhance self-concept in the classroom. Englewood Cliffs, New Jersey: Prentice Hall, 1976

Darling LAW. What do nurses want in a mentor? The Journal of Nursing Administration 1984; Oct: 42-44

Jung CG. Selected writings. (Ed. Start A.) London: Pan, 1983

Macquarrie J. Existentialism. Harmondsworth: Penquin, 1973

Rogers C. Client centred counselling. London: Constable, 1951

Shubin S. Burnout: the professional hazard in nursing. Nursing 1978; 18: 7

Singer P. Marx. Oxford: Oxford University Press, 1980

Storlie F. Burnout: the elaboration of a concept. American Journal of Nursing 1979; 79: 186-193

UKCC. Post-Registration Education and Practice. London: UKCC, 1995

Williams B. The problem of self. Cambridge: Cambridge University Press, 1973

Trust

The relationship that develops between a nurse and a patient or client is unique. Unlike the relationships in which an individual normally becomes involved, this relationship is one in which neither patient/client nor nurse has any real choice.

Apart from the situation where the individual engages a specific private nurse, the patient has no say as to who is selected to provide care. Equally, the nurse is rarely able to choose the patients allocated to her care or to opt out of involvement.

So the situation is one where two individuals who may have little or nothing in common socially (or in any other way) find themselves in an intimate interaction.

In addition, the nurse is likely to have access to information not normally disclosed to other people and to be involved in activities that breach customary social taboos. For example, in society it is not normal for an elderly male person to be seen naked by a female, except in a close family relationship. Older male patients who say wryly that 'the nurse is young enough to be my daughter' often remark upon the uniqueness of the situation. Similarly, the female patient is often embarrassed to be examined or cared for by a male doctor or nurse. The discomfort may not only be felt by the patient; some nurses feel uneasy in some situations, finding it difficult to separate normal social expectations from the interaction not only permitted but expected in intimate patient care. This situation still exists despite the changes that have occurred in recent years with many younger people being less embarrassed by nudity.

It is not only in the physical sphere that the relationship may be unusual. A ward will contain a wide range of individuals with different levels of education, with different occupations and from different social classes. There will also be a wide range of differences between patients in respect of personality type, values, beliefs, perceptions and personal preferences. However, as far as the nurse is concerned, these factors must make no difference to the way patients are treated or to the level of care that they receive.

In a small community, it is possible that the nurse may already know the patient, either personally or by virtue of the position they hold within the community. In this situation, it is vital that the nurse is able to detach herself from this personal knowledge, to ensure impartiality of care. Equally, any knowledge gained through the professional relationship must not be used outside the professional interaction.

COMMUNITY NURSING

Community nurses and health visitors have an additional privilege in that they are able to enter the homes of their clients. This will provide knowledge about the home that normally would only be acquired by chosen friends. Sometimes the patient or client's way of life will be such that the nurse may dislike or even disapprove of it. However, unless it has a bearing on the health of the patient, comment should not be made, nor should the conditions be related to other people.

The occupational health nurse has another concern: while her responsibility is the health and safety of the workforce, management may be anxious to receive information about the workers for organisational reasons. It may be difficult in some circumstances to separate what information is of a privileged nature, and therefore confidential, and what is of legitimate concern to management.

Often, when the relationship between the nurse and the patient is prolonged, a friendship over and above that of a professional relationship may develop. It is in this situation that the greatest care has to be taken to avoid abusing the relationship. It is important here to consider the power relationship that exists between nurse and patient. In almost all such relationships the nurse is necessarily in a dominant position vis-à-vis the patient. This is often due to the fact that the patient is dependent on the nurse; it is never the case that the nurse is dependent on the patient. Thus the relationship is never equal.

This unequal relationship may echo the earlier parent-child relationship and may be similar to what in psychotherapy is known as 'transference' (Procter, 1978; Schafer, 1983). When transference occurs in the nursing relationship, the patient comes to view the nurse as having all the positive qualities that were once seen in the father or mother. (This is 'positive' transference. In 'negative' transference the patient sees in the nurse all sorts of negative parental attributes. Fortunately in nursing negative transference is less common.) This unconscious mental process may lead to the patient becoming very dependent on the nurse. Examples of this happen when the patient clings to one nurse as being 'better' or 'more understanding' than other nurses. Such compliments are very flattering to the nurse, and are of course genuinely felt by the patient. All nurses need to be aware that this deeper level of dependence may occur and that it may bring with it the desire in the patient for a closer relationship with the nurse.

SAYING GOODBYE

It is particularly important for the longer-term nurse-patient relationship to be 'ended' gently and slowly by the nurse concerned. The process of saying 'goodbye' should be considered as soon as the nurse realises that the end of the relationship is in sight. Very often the patient who has become very dependent on the nurse will deny to herself that the relationship is going to end. In this case the patient will act as if the relationship will carry on indefinitely and will be very hurt by its ultimate ending. It is easy for the nurse to under-estimate how much the nurse-patient relationship can mean to the patient. It is vital, however, that the nurse can differentiate between a professional relationship and friendship. While it is tempting to think that there need be no differentiation between the two, and that patients and nurses can be 'friends', such a position fails to acknowledge the complex set of psychological processes that may be occurring when a dependent, often sick, person is meeting a 'care giver'. The relationship that develops out of these circumstances is usually very different from the circumstances that surround the more usual development of a friendship. In an ordinary friendship, the two people involved are usually of relatively equal status and are free to choose whether or not they become emotionally attached to each other. In the nurse-patient relationship, as we have seen, the two people involved do not informally 'choose' each other but find themselves together in a complex web of physical, emotional and social circumstances.

PSYCHIATRIC NURSING

In psychiatric nursing, the need to appreciate the boundaries of relationships is perhaps even more acute. The nature of the psychiatric nurse-patient relationship is such that the patient will often disclose to the nurse a considerable amount of their personal feelings and such disclosure can lead to dependence. It is important that the psychiatric nurse has a strong sense of her 'ego boundaries' – of the difference between her own identity and the identity of the patient. Thus, a degree of self-awareness is important here: through understanding something of our own make-up, we learn to discriminate between the other person and ourselves (Bond, 1986; Burnard, 1987). Without such awareness there is a danger of blurring the distinction between personal feelings and the feelings of the patient. Such blurring of roles and identities leads to confusion on the part of the patient and can lead to emotional exhaustion on the part of the nurse.

In the past, nurses were encouraged not to become emotionally involved with patients.

In recent years, the notion of being able to be totally objective in relationships has been called into question. Perhaps in the end it is a question of balance and of being able to judge the issue of therapeutic distance. If, on the one hand, the nurse stands too far back from the patient, she will be unable to empathise. In this case, she stands in what Martin Buber (1958) called an 'I-it' relationship to the patient: the patient is in danger of becoming an 'object', or a 'thing'. A classic example of how a patient may be turned into a 'thing' through this distancing is when a patient is referred to by diagnosis: 'the appendix in bed six'. If, however, the nurse stands too close, she may become so involved she will find it difficult to sort out her own emotions from those of the patient. The skill lies in establishing the optimum position at which to stand in relation to the patient: neither too involved nor too detached. This relationship Buber called the 'I-thou' relationship – one in which both parties meet as human beings. In everyday life, such emotional distances are extremely hard to judge, but the onus should be on the nurse to make the judgement.

MEDIA INTEREST

As has been already discussed in Chapter 5 on confidentiality, there may be particular problems if the patient is of interest to the press. While journalists have a job to do and readers thirst after details of celebrities' personal lives, it is the job of the nurse to ensure that no details are given to the media. For this reason, dealings with the media are best left to an authorised Press Officer. It is important that nurses, especially in public places such as buses or trains, do not indulge in what they may think is harmless gossip about who is in a ward, or any other details.

REWARDS

One of the methods that patients may use to try and equalise their relationship with the nurse is the giving of gifts. To many people it is a mystery why anyone enters nursing, and even more surprising that they stay, and assert that they would not do anything else! Not only does the nurse work unsocial hours and undertake hard physical work, she spends time with people who are at their least attractive due to illness, pain and distress. Some are aggressive and abusive, and monetary reward is relatively low. So where is the reward?

All people seek satisfaction in their daily life and this can be achieved in a variety of ways. It is quite common to speak of meeting the patients' needs, but nurses too have needs and it is the way in which these are, or are not, met that determines their level of satisfaction and whether they continue in the profession.

Social exchange

The meeting of needs is not restricted to nurses and social anthropologists have described the way needs are met as 'social exchange'. Cynics argue that little is done in the world from purely altruistic motives but that in every action there is a reward of some sort. While some aspects of social exchange have a complex economic connotation, other aspects appear to be important for their symbolic value and the social ties they produce. While studying a primitive society, Malinowski (1922) first described this situation by writing that there is

...a fundamental human impulse to display, to share, to bestow: the deep tendency to create social ties through the exchange of

gifts ... giving for the sake of giving is one of the most important features of Trobriand society and, from its very general and fundamental nature, I submit is a universal feature of all primitive societies.

A later writer, Levi-Strauss (1969) pointed out that even in Western society there is a strong feeling towards reciprocity which extends to invitations, Christmas cards and gifts and birthday presents; all of which by their exchange indicate social ties between giver and receiver. Gouldner (1969) also develops this idea and states that it would seem that there can be a stable pattern of reciprocity 'qua' exchange only insofar as each party has both rights and duties.

Homans (1961) considers that the process of exchange will only continue if both the participants derive some benefit from it.

The open secret of human exchange is to give to the other some behaviour that is more valuable to him than it is costly to you and to get from him some behaviour that is more valuable to you than it is costly to him.

The position within the UK health system is that it is considered 'free' because no payment is made at the point of delivery. As a result many patients feel that they get more care from the nurse than they have paid for, either by their insurance contributions or by the salary received by the nurse. In this case, the nurse is seen as the giver of the gift of care to the patient without the patient being able to reciprocate.

Indeed, there is no equality in the relationship between of the nurse and patient at the time care is being given. Although the patient may only be in a state of temporary dependence, in the case of the chronic sick, the handicapped or the dying patient, the dependence may be permanent. It is this inequality of relationship and the impossibility of reciprocity that places nursing in the category of occupations that are considered vocations, and gives nurses much of their esteem. However, in view of the reasons why individuals take up nursing, it may be that they are repaid by the dependency of the patient. Titmuss (1970) calls this type of activity 'creative altruism' – creative in that the self is satisfied with the help of others.

Social exchange in this context may be depicted as a balance: on one side the nurse's needs and on the other side the satisfaction provided by caring for patients or clients.

Patients rarely appreciate this situation and frequently say: 'How can I ever repay you, nurse?' – little realising that only by their being in the role of the patient can the role of the nurse exist. This inequality between the patient and the nurse may result in a feeling of stigma on behalf of the patient and it is to overcome this feeling that patients may offer the nurse some form of payment or gift.

While verbal gratitude is welcomed by nurses (indeed Stockwell (1976) found that nurses felt it was their right) the acceptance of gifts is more contentious. Section 7.4 of the Code states: 'You must refuse any gift or hospitality that might be interpreted, now or in the future, as an attempt to obtain preferential consideration.'

Most nurses are sensitive to the dangers of accepting gifts from patients but are less sensitive to accepting gifts from pharmaceutical companies or other firms. In this they are not alone; the medical profession frequently accepts hospitality from such sources. The question has to be asked: 'Does the acceptance of a diary or sponsorship of a conference put me or my organisation under any sort or pressure to buy from that firm in preference to any other?' If the answer is 'yes', then that offer must be refused.

Advertising

Section 7.1 of the Code emphasises that the nurse is in a very privileged position and must at all times act in such a way as to uphold the reputation of the profession, even when actions are not directly connected with professional practice.

Professional nurses are frequently asked, by friends and neighbours, for informal advice on healthcare matters. This is inevitable and can be seen as part of a nurse's contribution to society. Part of this advice may involve the nurse suggesting what medicine to take for a cough or how to feed a baby. In offering this advice it is likely that the nurse will mention a trade name. It is doubtful whether such advice could be considered as advertising. However, manufacturing firms may wish a nurse to endorse a specific product, either overtly, perhaps by appearing in an advertisement, or covertly, by offering free samples of products to be passed on to patients or clients. It is this type of activity that is referred to in the Code.

Advertising is an activity which aims to persuade people to act in a certain way and is a specific form of propaganda. There have been many studies investigating the way in which propaganda works. Katz and Lazarsfeld (1955) identified people who acted as 'opinion leaders'. These were the people whose opinion was sought by friends, neighbours and acquaintances. They also found that personal influence was more important than any other medium in producing change.

Peake (1955) showed that the effectiveness of information on attitude change was related to the importance of the outcome of the information on the individual. There are few areas of life more important to an individual than their health or the health of their family. These studies show the important role that may be held by health professionals in imparting information.

Nurses, midwives and health visitors are not only held in high regard and trust by the public but they have personal contact with many people and therefore any advice that they give is likely to be followed and, in the case of products, purchased. This places great responsibility on the shoulders of the nurse and means that any advice must be unbiased and based on the best possible knowledge.

Specialist nurses, that is, those dealing with a specific condition such as continence or asthma have a special responsibility to ensure that although they may be provided with a specific product to use in their place of work, patients and clients are made aware of alternatives.

To summarise, the registered nurse practitioner has a special place in society. The possession of the registered qualification implies not only the achievement of specific skills and knowledge, but also the holding of specific values and attitudes. This privileged status offered to members of the caring professions must not be abused and this requires high levels of behaviour in all areas of life. Most professionals accept this and act accordingly; however, not all appreciate the effect they may have on people by recommending particular products or the implication of acceptance of gifts from either firms or patients.

■ **QUESTIONS FOR REFLECTION AND DISCUSSION**

1 Do you feel in anyway inhibited by this element of the Code?

2 Should nurses be free to accept gifts from patients or firms?

REFERENCES

Bond M. Stress and self-awareness: a guide for nurses. London: Heinemann, 1986

Buber M. I and Thou. 2nd ed. New York: Scriber, 1958

Burnard P. Towards an epistemological basis for experiential learning in nurse education. Journal of Advanced Nursing 1987, 12: 189-193

Gouldner AW. The norm of reciprocity, a preliminary statement. American Sociological Review 1969; 28: 169

Homans GC. Social behaviour in its elementary forms. New York: Harcourt, Brace and World, 1961

Katz D, Lazarsfeld PF. Personal influence: the part played by people in the flow of mass communication. Glencoe: Free Press, 1955

Levi-Strauss C. The elementary structure of kindship. Boston: Beacon Press, 1969

Malinowski B. Argonauts of the Western Pacific. New York: Routledge and Kegan Paul ,1922

Peake H. Attitude and motivation. In: Jones MR (ed). Nebraska symposium on motivation. Lincoln: University of Nebraska Press, 1955

Proctor B. The counselling shop. London: Andre Deutsch, 1978

Schafer R. The analytical attitude. New York: Basic Books, 1983

Stockwell F. The unpopular patient. London: Heinemann, 1976

Titmuss R. The gift relationship. London: Allen and Unwin, 1970

8 Safety

To those who work in healthcare it comes as a great surprise to realise that there are people in the country who are very afraid of having to have attention from healthcare professionals. It is sometimes difficult to understand this fear – yet it may not be misplaced. Evidence exists that iatrogenic illness is a reality and it is sad, but true, that hospitals are dangerous places. In neither of these cases is the danger intentional, so the Clause 8 of the Code is apposite: 'As a registered nurse or midwife you must identify and minimise the risk to patients and clients.'

ENVIRONMENT OF CARE

Care may take place in a ward or department of a hospital or other institution, or in the individual's home. If the place of care is a clinical department of a hospital then the 'environment' will not only include the building, its furnishings and equipment, but the whole 'climate' of the unit and also the hospital. In this context, the word 'climate' refers to the attitudes of the staff, the interpersonal skills demonstrated by such staff and a whole range of almost subliminal factors, which bombard the patient as the consumer of care. Clearly the nurse has a part to play in producing the environment of care, which does not stop at clinical skills but includes the whole atmosphere in which those skills are applied. Most nurses are able to identify a 'happy' ward and patients are similarly sensitive to the atmosphere in which they find themselves.

Physical factors

It should be unnecessary to emphasise the importance of the appearance and cleanliness of the environment, but unfortunately in recent years these factors have become neglected. The advent and proliferation of antibiotics has bred a certain carelessness with regard to cleanliness in the most basic things and evidence exists which shows that staff do not regularly wash or disinfect their hands between caring for patients. The result of such behaviour is that some organisms have become antibiotic resistant. Patients thus infected have increased discomfort, delayed recovery with prolonged hospital stay, and in a few cases the results of the infection have been fatal. Cross-infection is also a very real danger and it is not unknown for a patient to enter hospital with one condition only to succumb to another.

There are other aspects of physical care, such as adequate ventilation, heating and lighting, which while not directly the responsibility of the nurse, should be monitored and the appropriate management informed if they fall below standard. Hunt and Sendell (1983), Du Gas (1983) and Faulkner (1985) all discuss in detail the importance of the physical aspects of care. Ethically, any failure in this regard is negligence. Paragraph 8.2 of the Code provides guidance, stating: 'Where you cannot remedy circumstances in the environment of care that could jeopardise standards of practice, you must report them to a senior person with sufficient authority to manage them and also, in the case of midwifery, to the supervisor of midwives. This must be supported by a written record.'

Psychological factors

The psychological effects of the climate of care are nebulous and less easy to describe. We all view the world from different perspectives and therefore the experience of illness will vary from person to person. It is dangerous to generalise about a person's psychological reaction to illness. George Kelly (1955), the personal construct psychologist, noted that 'if you want to know how someone feels, ask them, they might just tell you!' This may give a useful clue as to how to assess a patient's experience of what is occurring as care. Ask them, and continue to check with them as to how they are thinking and feeling.

A similar approach is useful in reading and applying psychological research in the field of nursing. It can never be the case that all research findings apply to all people, even if in similar situations to those studied in a specific research project. All that such research can do is offer a series of pointers. Research must be tested as to whether it applies or not to a particular person in their set of unique circumstances.

The same limitation must also apply to the social effects of the caring environment on the patient. For some people, ill health is merely a brief hiccup in their life experience. For others, any bout of illness, no matter how slight, is something of major concern. As you nurse, it is not appropriate to make value judgements on how the patient and the family deal with illness, but to note how they do, and to act accordingly. This refers back to the notion of sustained awareness alluded to in other sections of this book. It is only by constantly observing what patients are telling us that it is possible to make decisions as to how to help them. It is important to remember the cultural differences that may have an impact on how the environment of care is perceived (see Appendix 2).

Care at home

Although so far the discussion has been focused on care in hospital, the environment of care in a person's home will also impact on that patient's health. While the surroundings may be familiar to the person, it is likely that they may be perceived differently when the person becomes a patient. Once a person is designated as 'ill' by another family member they tend to be viewed differently by the family members and this will help amend their view of the home circumstances. The nurse will need to take these altered views into account when caring for a patient in their own home.

WORKING AS A TEAM

Chapter 4 discussed many of the aspects of working as a team member. In Section 8.2 the Code specifically refers to the need to protect patients and clients from any team member who may not be fit to practise 'for reasons of conduct, health or competence'.

Team loyalty often means that its members try to cover for any member of their team who is not functioning adequately. This is false loyalty – not only does it put the patients at risk, but also it does a disservice to the professional involved who also needs care and attention.

Aspects of personal behaviour which might in other spheres of employment remain the individual's private concern can give rise to doubts about their suitability to be involved in the care of others. Excessive use of alcohol, either when on duty or 'on call', may impair the individual's judgement leading to error. A similar situation may arise if the person is abusing drugs, whether from hospital supplies or privately. In both cases, if the person does not respond to an initial expression of concern, the matter must be reported to the appropriate hospital authority and the situation explained in writing.

A more difficult situation arises when it becomes obvious that an individual's competence is failing due to illness, either physical or psychological. The individual concerned may be desperately clinging on to their competence and employment by rationalising their situation, or they may have little or no insight into their deterioration. Great tact and sympathy is required in such cases, as the individual needs as much care as the patients need. Nevertheless, the prime concern is the safety of the patients and clients, and however sad the team may feel they must report the incompetent member. Occasionally the incompetence may be due to a lack of knowledge or skill. In this case remedial education is required and it must be made clear that until such action has been taken the person cannot be allowed access to patients.

Finally, there may be situations where the team member's behaviour is such that it can be classed as professional misconduct.

The management of the health organisation should instigate the first line of investigation and action, including possible temporary suspension from duty. Action will depend on the outcome of such an investigation.

In extreme cases, if the individual at fault takes no action, and none is instigated by management, then it may be the duty of the concerned team member to report the person to their professional body. If incompetence is reported to a professional statutory body, various steps may be taken. If the situation is deemed to be of immediate danger to patients, the professional's registration may be withdrawn at that point, prior to further investigation. This means that the person will be unable to continue in their employment. In some cases, following full investigation of the alleged incompetence or misconduct, restriction may be placed upon the person's practice. As an example, in a case of misuse of a drug the person may be banned from access to that drug. In more serious cases of professional misconduct the individual's registration is withdrawn. The individual has the right of appeal and following removal from the register may, after a suitable period of time, usually at least a year, apply for reinstatement. The statutory body will have to be certain that the conditions that led to removal from the register no longer exist and that the person has been rehabilitated. Over the years there has been considerable disquiet over the apparently varying standard of the decisions taken, not only between cases heard by a specific body but also between the controlling bodies of the different heathcare professions.

The body inquiring into the deaths of children undergoing heart surgery at Bristol recommended that there should be a rationalisation of this situation, saying: 'all health professionals should be subject to the same obligations as other healthcare professionals, including being subject to a regulatory body and a professional code of practice.' The inquiry also supported a national patient safety agency.

A previous chapter has dealt with 'whistle blowing' and a body has been set up by the Chief Medical Officer, called Organisation with a Memory. Its aim is to have an expert group learning from adverse events in the NHS in an open and non-punitive environment, with the aim of establishing a national database. This demonstrates not only that any one making a complaint will not be penalised, but also that anyone making a genuine mistake that might endanger a patient's life should feel able to own up to the matter without fear of disciplinary action. Healthcare professionals are human and despite their best efforts may sometimes make mistakes. It is important that these are investigated so that steps can be taken to prevent recurrence. Such steps may involve better education and training, more precise procedures and/or improved management, all aimed at improved patient safety.

This is 'clinical governance', and management is required by the Code (Paragraph 8.4) to 'have a duty of care towards patients and clients, colleagues, the wider community and the organisation in which you and your colleagues work. When facing professional dilemmas your first consideration in all activities must be the interests and safety of patients and clients.' It is not easy being a manager in the NHS with pressure being exerted by government targets, financial constraints, public expectations and clinical needs; however this aspect of the Code makes the prime responsibility quite clear and can be used a guideline when in difficulty. One of the interesting factors of the inquiry into the deaths of children at the Bristol Royal Infirmary was the fact that the Administrator, who was a registered medical practitioner but not working in the clinical field, had his registration removed. The General Medical Council found that, by not taking managerial action to halt inappropriate heart surgery, although he had been approached several times by concerned staff, he was guilty of professional misconduct.

RESOURCES

There are occasions when the safety of the patient or client is compromised not exclusively by staff but by the lack of resources. It is of little value to plan a specific aspect of care if the resources are not available to ensure its delivery. On the other hand, it may be considered negligent if the best level of care is not given because of ignorance as to the resources available. Nurses have a responsibility to make themselves aware of the facilities, agencies and healthcare policies of the workplace.

It is easy to blame lack of resources for poor care, but that is no excuse if the deficits have not been drawn to the attention of the appropriate manager.

Equipment that is not adequately maintained may also pose a threat to patient safety. Nurses have a reputation for 'making do', and while this may be an admirable quality in some situations it should not become routine behaviour. The Health and Safety at Work Act (1974) applies to healthcare establishments and most organisations have a committee responsible for implementation of its requirements.

EMERGENCY CARE

It is sometimes difficult to remember that once a person is on a professional register, then that fact will permeate the whole of their life, whether working in a professional role or as a private person. Nurses are used to being consulted by neighbours regarding health matters and most try to keep their profession a secret at parties or when on holiday, dreading the saga of health woes that may ensue if their status becomes known. Although it might be tempting, as in the story of the Good Samaritan, to 'pass by on the other side' when confronted by an accident or illness in a public place most nurses accept that there is a responsibility to give what assistance may be required. Paragraph 8.5 of the Code states: 'In an emergency, in or outside the work setting, you have a professional duty to provide care. The care provided would be judged against what could reasonably be expected from someone with your knowledge, skills and abilities when placed in those particular circumstances.'

This is a comforting statement, as many nurses feel incompetent outside the familiar setting of the hospital with its equipment. Also, in this era of increasing litigation there is always the spectre of the lawyer questioning whether it was 'reasonable care'. To ensure against misunderstanding, the NMC have defined what is meant by 'reasonable care in this context. They quote the case of Bolam v Friern Hospital Management Committee (1957) which produced the following definition:

The test is the standard of the ordinary skilled man exercising and professing to have special skill. A man need not possess the highest expert skill at the risk of being found negligent ... it is enough that he exercises the skill of an ordinary man exercising that particular art.

This definition has been supported and clarified in a subsequent case, Bolitho v City and Hackney Health Authority (1993).

ENSURING SAFETY

Following the discussion in this section it becomes clear that to ensure the safety of patients or clients the nurse must possess knowledge and skill, as well as an appreciation of the facts of any given situation, awareness of current health and safety standards and probably a degree of political awareness. It is important to be able to question why certain standards of conduct and safety exist. It is tempting to believe that all such standards arise from rational decisions made on current research and theory. In the ideal world this would probably be the case, but in reality, such decisions are placed upon much shakier foundations, including tradition, political expediency, changing ideologies of healthcare, consumer expectations and even sometimes on the basis of crisis management. On many occasions, decisions about standards are made after an incident of failure of care has occurred. This is retrospective policy formation and unless based on sound enquiry and research may only result in 'shutting the stable door after the horse has gone'. Useful discussions about political issues in care are dealt with by Salvage (1985) and Clay (1987).

■ QUESTIONS FOR REFLECTION AND DISCUSSION

1 In your place of work, do you know the steps to take if you are concerned about any aspect of a patient's safety?

2 How can you become aware of workplace policies of care?

3 What power do you have to affect healthcare practice?

REFERENCES

Clay T. Nurses, power and politics. London: Heinemann, 1987

Du Gas BW. Introduction to patient care. A comprehensive approach to nursing. 4th ed. Philadelphia: WB Saunders, 1983

Faulkner A. Nursing: a creative approach. London: Baillière Tindall, 1985

Hunt P, Sendell B. Nursing the adult with specific physiological disturbance. Basingstoke: Macmillan, 1983

Kelly G. The psychology of personal constructs: Vols. 1, 2. New York: Merton, 1955

Ministry of Health. Inquiry into Bristol Royal Infirmary. London: HMSO, 2000

Salvage J. The politics of nursing. London: Heinemann, 1985

9 Conclusion

In the preceding chapters we have offered a variety of theories and practical approaches to ethical and professional issues in nursing. In one sense, how we decide to act in a nursing situation is determined for us by the Code of Conduct. The Code lays down broad principles and offers a framework to guide professional action. What we as individuals have to do, however, is to interpret those principles – often we have to decide for ourselves what to do. This book has also offered some pointers to how such decisions may be made. The book cannot make those decisions. Nor can it account for the many and varied situations that arise in everyday nursing practice that are exceptions to the rule; after all, in real life, situations are rarely experienced as they are portrayed in books! In closing, it may be worth reconsidering some of the ways of making ethical and professional decisions that have been alluded to in this book.

CODES

First, we may appeal to a code of conduct as a means of decision making. Clearly, as this book is about such a code, it is felt that codes can be a useful means of helping and guiding the decision-making process. There are, of course, other codes of practice that can be referred to, the most notable being particular ethical codes as outlined within specific religious groups. We have noted, too, that agnostics and atheists may also have codes to which they may refer.

CONSCIENCE

Another means of making ethical and professional decisions is through consideration of conscience. Freud called the person's conscience their 'superego' and argued that its development evolved from the internalisation of parental values, beliefs and attitudes at an early age (Hall, 1954). Thus when we appeal to our conscience it is as though we were experiencing one or both of our parents 'looking over our shoulder' as we make a particular decision. Another way of viewing the development of conscience is to see it in terms of socialisation. As a person grows and develops through life he not only absorbs and learns the particular set of beliefs and values of his parents but also takes into account the broader set of beliefs and values of the particular culture in which he lives and is raised. This process of socialisation must clearly exert an effect upon the way the individual makes decisions. Decisions are not made in isolation, nor can they be made outside the culture in which the individual lives. Lives are lived and decisions made in the context of the society in which the individual dwells.

This notion of culture-bound ethical and professional decision making is important. It is tempting to think that the beliefs and values of our culture are the 'right' ones. Clearly, different cultures produce different values, and different values will be reflected in different sorts of ethical and professional decisions.

UTILITARIANISM

Another approach to ethical and professional decision making is via the notion of utilitarianism, arguing that what is good and right is the decision which creates the greatest happiness for the greatest number of people. Indeed, many decisions are made on this basis, but we may want to ponder upon the question of who decides what is likely to create the greatest good, and what happens to those who are not contained within the greatest number.

It may also be worth considering Sartre's (1956,1973) notion of 'situational ethics'. In order to understand this notion it is important to consider the theory of existentialism, for which Sartre was famous.

EXISTENTIALISM

Existentialism, as an approach to philosophy, may be encapsulated by Sartre's famous epigram that 'existence comes prior to essence' (Sartre, 1973 p. 26). In order to understand this, it may be useful to look at an example that Sartre himself uses. If we consider a man-made object, such as a paperknife, we can realise that before it came into existence, someone sat down and designed it. For the paperknife, then, its 'essence' came prior to its 'existence': before it was made, someone had a fair idea what it was going to be for. Sartre argues that, for people, exactly the opposite is true. First of all we 'exist', then we create our 'essence'. There is no one 'designing' before we exist. We start from nothing and then we are responsible for what we become.

Contained in Sartre's argument is the notion that people are (psychologically, at least) free to choose how they view themselves and the world. There is often a temptation for people to blame the past, other people, or circumstances for how they are today. While these factors clearly have an influence, Sartre is saying that today the individual can decide for himself: he can choose to blame the past or circumstances, but that does not change his personal responsibility for how he decides to behave. A person is what he makes himself. Clearly, as we have noted, this is a psychological freedom – a freedom of thought. We cannot exercise a similar physical or social freedom. It would be ludicrous, for instance, to argue that a person could choose to be seven feet tall or that he could choose the social circumstances into which he was born! The point that Sartre is making is that, given those physical and social limitations, people are makers of their own destiny.

It may be noted at this point that while Sartre's view of existentialism is atheistic, this need not necessarily be the case. Other commentators have argued for a Christian existentialism (Macquarrie, 1966). This version argues that while God is the creator, man still has to decide on his own future and make his own decisions. God has given man 'free will'. In Sartre's version, God does not exist in the first place: man has free will anyway.

The second issue is the individual's responsibility for his own life and decision making. A person cannot claim freedom and not acknowledge responsibility. Imagine, for instance, that I say 'I am free to get married and have chosen to do so, but the decision is really my parents'.' Such a statement is clearly illogical. If I am free to choose, I cannot make another person responsible for my choice, otherwise no such choice exists.

These factors have important implications for ethical and professional decision making. If Sartre's position is accepted (and it may not be) then the responsibility for all decisions rests squarely on the shoulders of the individual.

It may be worth considering to what extent nursing situations can be clarified through an appeal to situational ethics. In many situations the nurse is dependent on others to share in making decisions. Nor may we take on Sartre's notion of total responsibility. Such argument can, however, make the nurse aware of how important ethical and professional decisions are, and how important it is for her to shoulder responsibility. Such arguments can also awaken nurses to the importance of considering the context of ethical decision making. While the Code of Conduct can be used as a guide to such decisions, it must also be borne in mind that this situation, for this person, is unique. It is necessary to remain open-minded and flexible and, where possible, come to each situation afresh. In weighing up the pros and cons of any situation and relating them to prior experience and knowledge, it must also be acknowledged how different each situation is.

PAST EXPERIENCE

Perhaps, however, Sartre's position is a little 'black and white'. It can be argued that many ethical and professional decisions are made by considering the evidence and comparing that evidence with previous situations. Out of this consideration and reflection on past experience the 'new' decision is made. An example may be useful here. If a nurse manager is attempting to make an important decision as to how to best advise a member of staff, she may well reflect back to previous situations which mirror this one, consider the 'unique' features of the present situation and look for some sort of 'fit' between the past and present experience. Out of this balanced view, the manager makes her decision. In one sense she is alone in making that decision. In another sense, however, she has considerable precedent, in terms of her own and other people's past experience, on which to draw. Decisions are never made in isolation. As has been discussed throughout this book, they arise out of a wide range of cultural, social, psychological and personal contexts. Perhaps 'unique' situations are not as unique as they first appear!

One particular theme has recurred frequently throughout this book; the notion of a 'golden rule'. This is usually expressed as the idea that we should treat others as we ourselves would wish to be treated. This would seem to be a necessary requirement for anyone who makes ethical and professional decisions. The emphasis is the importance of fundamental human considerations: respect for others, consideration of the possible consequences of action, and the need always to treat people as subjects, never as objects. Without such fundamental considerations, it is difficult to see how ethical and professional decisions can begin to be made. It is notable, however, that even the 'golden rule' has its limitations. It may work well enough all of the time that the individual is a thoughtful, caring person who wishes themselves to be treated that way. It does not account for the person who does not care how they are treated! In this case, the notion of treating others as you would wish to be treated does not apply. Christians, of course, quote a higher authority for this type of action, the words of Jesus: 'This is my commandment, that ye love one another...' (John 15:12).

This book offers a variety of ways of addressing ethical and professional issues. The subject is a complex one and we hope that the book has raised more questions than it has attempted to answer. There cannot be a ready-made guide to the issues raised, nor can there be a consensus on how to make decisions. What all ethical and professional decisions require is a firm grasp of as many of the facts as possible, an understanding of the various philosophical and theoretical ways of addressing problems of this nature, plus a certain courage and determination to make decisions. This is true all the fields of nursing, from the learner to the most senior nurse administrator or educator. Nursing is necessarily about decision making.

Ethics and professional practice are constantly changing. Advances in medical science such as the human genome project, transplant surgery, fertilisation programmes and issues regarding creating life (cloning) and hastening death (euthanasia) inevitably have implications for nurses and require fresh thinking and decisions about involvement. The ideas in this book offer ways of thinking about situations, contexts and people. What can never be offered is a final, authoritative answer to all the issues that may arise. The important thing as a nurse is to develop and remain a reflective practitioner: a person who thinks and reflects about what he or she does and acts knowingly.

REFERENCES

Hall C. A primer of Freudian psychology. New York: Basic Books, 1954

Macquarrie J. Studies in Christian existentialism. London: SCM, 1966

Sartre J-P. Being and nothingness: essay on phenomenological ontology. (Trans. Barnes H.) New York: Philosophical Library, 1956

Sartre J-P. Existentialism and humanism. (Trans. Mairet P.) London: Methuen, 1973

Appendix 1
Code of Professional Conduct

As a registered nurse, midwife or health visitor, you are personally accountable for your practice. In caring for patients and clients, you must:

- respect the patient or client as an individual

- obtain consent before you give any treatment or care

- protect confidential information

- co-operate with others in the team

- maintain your professional knowledge and competence

- be trustworthy

- act to identify and minimise risk to patients and clients.

These are the shared values of all the United Kingdon health care regulatory bodies.

1 Introduction

1.1   The purpose of the *Code of professional conduct* is to:

- inform the professions of the standard of professional conduct required of them in the exercise of their professional accountability and practice

- inform the public, other professions and employers of the standard of professional conduct that they can expect of a registered practitioner.

1.2   As a registered nurse, midwife or health visitor, you must:

- protect and support the health of individual patients and clients

- protect and support the health of the wider community

- act in such a way that justifies the trust and confidence the public have in you

- uphold and enhance the good reputation of the professions.

1.3   You are personally responsible for your practice. This means that you are answerable for your actions and omissions, regardless of advice or directions from another professional.

1.4   You have a duty of care to your patients and clients, who are entitled to receive safe and competent care.

1.5   You must adhere to the laws of the country in which you are practising.

2 As a registered nurse, midwife or health visitor, you must respect the patient or client as an individual

2.1   You must recognise and respect the role of patients and clients as partners in their care and the contribution they can make to it. This involves identifying their preferences regarding care and respecting these within the limits of professional practice, existing legislation, resources and the goals of the therapeutic relationship.

2.2   You are personally accountable for ensuring that you promote and protect the interests and dignity of patients and clients, irrespective of gender, age, race, ability, sexuality, economic status, lifestyle, culture and religious or political beliefs.

2.3   You must, at all times, maintain appropriate professional boundaries in the relationships you have with patients and clients. You must ensure that all aspects of the relationship focus exclusively upon the needs of the patient or client.

2.4   You must promote the interests of patients and clients. This includes helping individuals and groups gain access to health and social care, information and support relevant to their needs.

2.5   You must report to the relevant person or authority, at the earliest possible time, any conscientious objection that may be relevant to your professional practice. You must continue to provide care to the best of your ability until alternative arrangements are implemented.

3 As a registered nurse, midwife or health visitor, you must obtain consent before you give any treatment or care

3.1   All patients and clients have the right to receive information about their condition. You must be sensitive to their needs and respect the wishes of those who refuse or are unable to receive information about their condition. Information should be accurate, truthful and presented in such a way as to make it easily understood. You may need to seek legal or professional advice, or guidance from your employer, in relation to the giving or withholding of consent.

3.2 You must respect patients' or clients' autonomy – their right to decide whether or not to undergo any health care intervention – even where a refusal may result in harm or death to themselves or a foetus, unless a court of law orders to the contrary. This right is protected in law, although in circumstances where the health of the foetus would be severely compromised by any refusal to give consent, it would be appropriate to discuss this matter fully within the team, and possibly to seek external advice and guidance (see clause 4).

3.3 When obtaining valid consent, you must be sure that it is:

● given by a legally competent person

● given voluntarily

● informed.

3.4 You should presume that every patient and client is legally competent unless otherwise assessed by a suitably qualified practitioner. A patient or client who is legally competent can understand and retain treatment information and can use it to make an informed choice.

3.5 Those who are legally competent may give consent in writing, orally or by co-operation. They may also refuse consent. You must ensure that all your discussions and associated decisions relating to obtaining consent are documented in the patient's or client's health care records.

3.6 When patients or clients are no longer legally competent and thus have lost the capacity to consent to or refuse treatment and care, you should try to find out whether they have previously indicated preferences in an advance statement. You must respect any refusal of treatment or care given when they were legally competent, providing that the decision is clearly applicable to the present circumstances and that there is no reason to believe that they have changed their minds. When such a statement is not available, the patients' or clients' wishes, if known, should be taken into account. If these wishes are not known, the criteria for treatment must be that it is in their best interests.

3.7   The principles of obtaining consent apply equally to those people who have a mental illness. Whilst you should be involved in their assessment, it will also be necessary to involve relevant people close to them; this may include a psychiatrist. When patients and clients are detained under statutory powers (mental health acts), you must ensure that you know the circumstances and safeguards needed for providing treatment and care without consent.

3.8   In emergencies where treatment is necessary to preserve life, you may provide care without patients' or clients' consent, if they are unable to give it, provided you can demonstrate that you are acting in their best interests.

3.9   No-one has the right to give consent on behalf of another competent adult. In relation to obtaining consent for a child, the involvement of those with parental responsibility in the consent procedure is usually necessary, but will depend on the age and understanding of the child. If the child is under the age of 16 in England and Wales, 12 in Scotland and 17 in

Northern Ireland, you must be aware of legislation and local protocols relating to consent.

3.10 Usually the individual performing a procedure should be the person to obtain the patient's or client's consent. In certain circumstances, you may seek consent on behalf of colleagues if you have been specially trained for that specific area of practice.

3.11 You must ensure that the use of complementary or alternative therapies is safe and in the interests of patients and clients. This must be discussed with the team as part of the therapeutic process and the patient or client must consent to their use.

4 As a registered nurse, midwife or health visitor, you must co-operate with others in the team

4.1 The team includes the patient or client, the patient's or client's family, informal carers and health and social care professionals in the National Health Service, independent and voluntary sectors.

4.2 You are expected to work co-operatively within teams and to respect the skills, expertise and contributions of your colleagues. You must treat them fairly and without discrimination.

4.3 You must communicate effectively and share your knowledge, skill and expertise with other members of the team as required for the benefit of patients and clients.

4.4 Health care records are a tool of communication within the team. You must ensure that the health care record for the patient or client is an accurate account of treatment, care planning and delivery. It should be consecutive, written with the involvement of the patient or client wherever practicable and completed as soon as possible after an event has occurred. It should provide clear evidence of the care planned, the decisions made, the care delivered and the information shared.

4.5 When working as a member of a team, you remain accountable for your professional conduct, any care you provide and any omission on your part.

4.6 You may be expected to delegate care delivery to others who are not registered nurses or midwives. Such delegation must not compromise existing care but must be directed to meeting the needs and serving the interests of patients and clients. You remain accountable for the appropriateness of the delegation, for ensuring that the person who does the work is able to do it and that adequate supervision or support is provided.

4.7 You have a duty to co-operate with internal and external investigations.

5 As a registered nurse, midwife or health visitor, you must protect confidential information

5.1 You must treat information about patients and clients as confidential and use it only for the purposes for which it was given. As it is impractical to obtain consent every time you need to share information with others, you should ensure that patients and clients understand that some information may be made available to other members of the team involved in the delivery of care. You must guard against breaches of confidentiality by protecting information from improper disclosure at all times.

5.2 You should seek patients' or clients' wishes regarding the sharing of information with their family and others. When a patient or client is considered incapable of giving permission, you should consult with relevant colleagues.

5.3 If you are required to disclose information outside the team that will have personal consequences for patients or clients, you must obtain their consent. If the patient or client withholds consent, or if consent cannot be obtained for whatever reason, disclosures may be made only where:

- they can be justified in the public interest (usually where disclosure is essential to protect the patient or client or someone else from the risk of significant harm)

- They are required by law or by the order of a court.

5.4 Where there is an issue of child protection, you must act at all times in accordance with national and local policies.

6 As a registered nurse, midwife or health visitor, you must maintain your professional knowledge and competence

6.1 You must keep your knowledge and skills up-to-date throughout your working life. In particular, you should take part regularly in learning activities that develop your competence and performance.

6.2   To practise competently, you must possess the knowledge, skills and abilities required for lawful, safe and effective practice without direct supervision. You must acknowledge the limits of your professional competence and only undertake practice and accept responsibilities for those activities in which you are competent.

6.3   If an aspect of practice is beyond your level of competence or outside your area of registration, you must obtain help and supervision from a competent practitioner until you and your employer consider that you have acquired the requisite knowledge and skill.

6.4   You have a duty to facilitate students of nursing, midwifery and health visiting and others to develop their competence.

6.5   You have a responsibility to deliver care based on current evidence, best practice and, where applicable, validated research when it is available.

7 As a registered nurse, midwife or health visitor, you must be trustworthy

7.1   You must behave in a way that upholds the reputation of the professions. Behaviour that compromises this reputation may call your registration into question even if it is not directly connected to your professional practice.

7.2   You must ensure that your registration status is not used in the promotion of commercial products or services, declare any financial or other interests in relevant organisations providing such goods or services and ensure that your professional judgement is not influenced by any commercial considerations.

7.3   When providing advice regarding any product or service relating to your professional role or area of practice, you must be aware of the risk that, on account of your professional title or qualification, you could be perceived by the patient or client as endorsing the product. You should fully explain the advantages and disadvantages of alternative products so that the patient or client can make an informed choice. Where you recommend a specific product, you must ensure that your advice is based on evidence and is not for your own commercial gain.

7.4   You must refuse any gift, favour or hospitality that might be interpreted, now or in the future, as an attempt to obtain preferential consideration.

7.5   You must neither ask for nor accept loans from patients, clients or their relatives and friends.

8 As a registered nurse, midwife or health visitor, you must act to identify and minimise the risk to patients and clients

8.1   You must work with other members of the team to promote health care environments that are conducive to safe, therapeutic and ethical practice.

8.2   You must act quickly to prevent patients and clients from risk if you have good reason to believe that you or a colleague, from your own or another profession, may not be fit to practise for reasons of conduct, health or competence. You should be aware of the terms of legislation that offer protection for people who raise concerns about health and safety issues.

8.3   Where you cannot remedy circumstances in the environment of care that could jeopardise standards of practice, you must report them to a senior person with sufficient authority to manage them and also, in the case of midwifery, to the supervisor of midwives. This must be supported by a written record.

8.4   When working as a manager, you have a duty of care towards patients and clients, colleagues, the wider community and the organisation in which you and your colleagues work. When facing professional dilemmas, your first consideration in all activities must be the interests and safety of patients and clients.

8.5   In an emergency, in or outside the work setting, you have a professional duty to provide care. The care provided would be judged against what could reasonably be expected from someone with your knowledge, skills and abilities when placed in those particular circumstances.

Glossary

Accountable   Responsible for something or to someone.

Care   To provide help or comfort.

Competent   Possessing the skills and abilities required for lawful, safe and effective professional practice without direct supervision.

Patient and client   Any individual or group using a health service.

Reasonable   The case of *Bolam v Friern Hospital Management Committee* (1957) produced the following definition of what is reasonable.
'The test is the standard of the ordinary skilled man exercising and professing to have that special skill. A man need not possess the highest expert skill at the risk of being found negligent... it is sufficient if he exercises the skill of an ordinary man exercising that particular art.'
This definition is supported and clarified by the case of *Bolitho v City and Hackney Health Authority* (1993).

This *Code of professional conduct* was published by the Nursing and Midwifery Council in April 2002 and came into effect on 1 June 2002.

Reproduced with permission of the Nursing and Midwifery Council

Appendix 2
Cultural Variations

DOS AND DON'TS RELATING TO VARIOUS CULTURES (D COOPER 1992)

Name

Don't use Western titles, such as Mr, Mrs, Miss, Ms.

Don't ask non-Christians for a Christian name.

Do ask for a family name or first name.

Do avoid repetitions in clinical notes. Find the correct family name first rather than misuse several different names.

Language

Don't assume that all ethnic minority groups speak English.

Don't assume that all ethnic minority groups do not speak English.

Do avoid making assumptions by using accurate assessment procedures.

Don't use the family to interpret intimate questions.

Don't use a family member to break bad news. He or she may avoid the issue if it is believed to be too stressful for the client.

Do use an interpreter who understands medical terminology, this will avoid stress for the interpreter and client and also avoid misinterpretation.

Do be aware that only women may ask intimate questions of women in some cultures. This will avoid wrong information being passed, and avoid embarrassment.

Religion

Don't generalise about a client's religion.

Do remember that for Buddhists, Christians, Jews, Sikhs, Hindus and Muslims, religion may be an integral part of daily life.

Do avoid incorrect assumptions; find out the different beliefs and approaches.

Do record clearly and make notes of the client's wishes to see or have present a representative from his religion.

Do ask the family who you should contact if the client is not able to relay this to you.

Do remember that many Eastern religions fast on certain days; pray at certain times; wear religious objects or symbols.

Don't mistake religious objects or symbols for jewellery.

Do check to see if any nursing interventions will compromise any religious beliefs.

Do inform the client and/or family of any nursing interventions before commencing, to check religious beliefs.

Do check religious observations with client and family.

Do consult religious advisors or teachers to gain permission and/or to obtain exemption, to allow procedures to take place. Ensure she explains this to the client.

Diet

Don't give Jews or Muslims pork or pork products.

Do make sure that other meat offered to Muslims has been naturally slaughtered by the halal method.

Do remember that not all Jewish people eat kosher food (specially prepared to make pure).

Do remember that not all Muslims eat halal meat.

Do consult the client regarding any diet preferences.

Do remember that meal times are family occurrences in Eastern culture; matters relating to the family are often discussed here.

Do remember that being taken out of a close family environment can be frightening and cause loneliness, which may cause loss of appetite.

Do invite the family to bring in food and to join in meal times, if at all possible and practicable.

Personal hygiene

Do remember that to Sikhs, Hindus and Muslims washing in still water is considered unclean.

Do supply the client with a jug of water and a bowl and/or a running tap and empty washbasin to allow hand, face and body washing.

Do make exceptions if the client is dependent.

Do remember that Muslims use the right hand for eating and food preparation, and the left hand for cleaning themselves and other procedures. Anyone unable to do this because of injury or other health reasons will need counselling and discussion relating to ways of surmounting the problem, (it may be useful to supply a plastic glove).

Modesty

Don't compromise the client's dignity and modesty.

Do remember that exposure of the female body to the male will cause distress in certain cultures, especially if the client is in purdah (the duration of menstruation).

Do offer separate bays in mixed-bedded wards, or if possible a single room, especially for those in purdah.

Do remember that hospital gowns often expose more than they cover, and are therefore unacceptable.

Do avoid exposure of arms or legs; for example, in the case of a fractured limb. Do additional covering to protect modesty.

Skin and hair

Do remember that Afro hair may be brittle and dry; add moisturiser or oil to the scalp and comb regularly.

Do remember to ask the client what they use for skin moisturising.

Do remember that dark-skinned people are prone to keloid scarring (hyperkeratinisation); invasive treatment will cause excessive pigmented scarring.

Do remember to inject or undertake invasive procedures in a site that will avoid disfigurement if possible.

Don't assume that children of Asian, African or Southern European descent have bruising if you see marks around the sacrum, buttocks, or hand and wrist; these may be Mongolian blue spots.

Do avoid accusations of child abuse by undertaking full and proper assessment and advice.

Hospital procedures

Do give careful thought to hospital procedures and routines before commencing them.

Do remember that discussing elimination or other intimate health issues may be culturally offensive.

Do approach all patients sensitively, ensure privacy and maintain the individual's right to self-respect.

Do remember that some medications and treatments may be taboo for some religious groups.

Don't give Jehovah's Witnesses blood transfusions.

Don't give Muslims, Jews and vegetarians iron injections derived from pigs.

Don't give insulin of porcine origin to Jews or Muslims.

Do remember that many emollients contain animal derivatives.

Do remember that some medications have an alcohol base which may be forbidden in some cultural groups. The client with a drinking problem may wish to avoid these preparations.

Do be aware of all preparations likely to contain potentially taboo or offensive ingredients.

Visiting

Do remember that limiting visiting to two people may cause distress in extended family cultures.

Do remember that West Indian, Asian and Middle Eastern families like to visit as a family.

Do remember that the 'family' may include children, uncles, aunts, grandchildren, parents and grandparents.

Do compromise over visiting, and numbers visiting per bed.

Do remember that open visiting can be more accommodating.

Do allow the family to participate in the client's care.

Myths

Don't believe that people from different races have low pain thresholds. This is not true; for example:

Japanese may smile or laugh when in pain, thus avoiding loss of face.

Anglo-Saxons may be sullen and withdrawn, portraying the stiff-upper lip image.

Eastern Europeans, Greeks and Italians express pain vocally and freely.

Do remember that every individual has a different level of pain tolerance, regardless of race, culture, country of origin or creed.

Death and bereavement

Do involve client and family in the care.

Do remember that Eastern cultures like to take an active part in the care of dying relatives, especially last offices.

Do remember that in certain cultures, custom and practice will need to be followed if the client is to proceed along the continuum of life following her earthly death.

Do ensure that you are conversant with specific cultural requirements for death, bereavement and last offices.

Don't deny the family the right to participate in last offices as this will increase the pain already being experienced and may slow down the grieving process.

Do negotiate to minimise anxiety and allow some participation, when the family's wishes come into conflict with hospital policies and procedures. This will assist the grieving process.

Do compromise – the client and family have only one chance to say their goodbyes.

Cooper D, reproduced from Wright H and Giddey M (1992) Mental Health Nursing: From First Principles to Professional Practice. London: Chapman and Hall, with permission

Recommended Further Reading

Baruth LG. An introduction to the counseling profession. Englewood Cliffs, New Jersey: Prentice-Hall, 1987

Beauchamp TL, Childress JF. Principles of biomedical ethics. 4th ed. New York: Oxford University Press, 1994

Beardshaw V. Conscientious objectors at work. London: Social Audit Ltd, 1981

Benner P, Wrubel J. The primacy of caring. Menlo Park, California: Addison Wesley, 1989

Berry C. The rites of life: Christians and bio-medical decision making. London: Hodder and Stoughton, 1987

Bok S. Lying: moral choice in public and private life. London: Quartet, 1980

Brazier M. Medicine: patients and the law. Harmondsworth: Pelican, 1987

British Medical Association. Handbook of medical ethics. London: BMA, 1980

British Medical Association. Advanced statements about medical treatments. London: BMA, 1995

British Medical Association. Withholding and withdrawing life-prolonging medical treatment: guidance for decision making. London: BMA/BMJ Books, 1999

Campbell AV. Moral dilemmas in medicine. 3rd ed. Edinburgh: Churchill Livingstone, 1984

Chambliss DF. Beyond caring: hospitals, nurses and the social organisation of ethics. Chicago: University of Chicago Press, 1996

Davis BD (ed). Research into nurse education. London: Croom Helm, 1983

Department of Health. The patients' charter and you. London: Department of Health 1992

Department of Health. Being heard: the report of a review committee on NHS complaints procedures. London: Department of Health, 1994

Dimond B. Patients' rights, responsibilities and the nurse. 2nd ed. Salisbury: Quay Books, 1999

Dimond B. Legal aspects of nursing. 3rd ed. Oxford: Pearson Education, 2001

Downie RS, Calman KC. Healthy respect: ethics in health care. London: Faber and Faber, 1987

Doxiadis S (ed). Ethical dilemmas in health promotion. Chichester: Wiley, 1987

Evans B. Freedom to choose. London: The Bodley Head, 1984

Gillon R. Philosophical medical ethics. Chichester: Wiley, 1986

Harris J. The value of life: an introduction to medical ethics. London: Routledge and Kegan Paul, 1986

Johnstone MJ. Bioethics: a nursing perspective. 2nd ed. Marrickville, New South Wales: WB Saunders, 1994

Kleinman A. The illness narrative: suffering, healing and the human condition. New York: Basic Books, 1988

McGilloway O, Myco E (eds). Nursing and spiritual care. London: Harper Row, 1984

Neuberger J. Caring for people of different faiths. London: Austin Cornish, 1987

Papper S. Doing right: everyday medical ethics. Boston: Little,Brown, 1983

Roach Sr. MS. The human act of caring: a blueprint for the health professions. Ottawa, Ontario: Canadian Hospital Association, 1987

Sampson C. The neglected ethic: religious and cultural factors in the care of patients. London: McGraw-Hill, 1982

Tadd W (ed). Ethics in nursing education, research and management. Basingstoke: Palgrave McMillan, 2002

Tschudin V. Ethics in nursing: the caring relationship. 3rd ed. Oxford: Elsevier Science, 2003

Tschudin V (ed). Approaches to ethics: nursing beyond boundaries. Oxford: Elsevier Science, 2003

Index